HOW TO USE A MEDICAL LIBRARY
Seventh Edition

HOW TO USE A MEDICAL LIBRARY
Seventh Edition

Leslie T. Morton FLA
*Formerly Librarian, National Institute
for Medical Research*

and

Derek J. Wright BA, ALA, MIInfSc
*Formerly Librarian, British Medical
Association*

CLIVE BINGLEY LONDON

© L.T. Morton and D.J. Wright 1990

Published by
Library Association Publishing Ltd
7 Ridgmount Street
London WC1E 7AE

First edition published by Heinemann 1934
Sixth edition published by Heinemann 1979
This seventh edition published by
Library Association Publishing Ltd 1990

British Library Cataloguing in Publication Data
Morton, Leslie T.
  How to use a medical library – 7th ed.
  1. Medicine. Information sources
  I. Title II. Wright, Derek J.
  610'.7

ISBN 0-85157-466-1

Typeset from author's disk in 11/12 pt Garamond
by Saxon Printing Ltd, Derby.
Printed and made in Great Britain by Redwood Press Ltd,
Melksham, Wilts.

CONTENTS

1 Introduction

Progress in medical science is dependent upon experiment and research, in which the part played by the library is comparable in importance to that of the laboratory. No responsible research worker is entitled to advance what he believes to be a new theory until he has explored the existing literature on the subject; nor should he embark upon experimental study until he has ascertained what has already been achieved or attempted on the same or related subjects.

The quality of medical research depends largely upon the efficient exchange of information. It is essential, therefore, that medical literature should be easily and rapidly accessible to practitioners and research workers and that they in turn should be able to use it to full advantage.

However, although the literature of medicine is most efficiently indexed and abstracted, the researcher or student does not always make full use of it. In the better libraries he is given unrestricted access to the literature; he is encouraged to help himself and should learn how to do so.

Over the last 25 years the introduction of computer technology has produced dramatic changes in medical and other libraries. It has made possible the generation of databases – machine-readable data banks of bibliographical information – that can be searched in a matter of minutes, in contrast to the hours spent in searching by hand. The modern medical library is now equipped with a computer terminal that can be linked 'online' by telephone to various databases located elsewhere, and modern librarians are trained to carry out sophisticated and complex literature searches. More recently the introduction of CD-ROM (Compact Disk – Read-Only Memory) has provided databases that the reader can search for himself.

1

Many library catalogues are now available online, and most libraries at least have a terminal to search remote databases. Microcomputers can also be used for a variety of library housekeeping routines and for the production of letters, leaflets, bibliographies and other printed matter.

Some medical libraries offer formal instruction and/or provide guides to readers in the use of the library. One of the objectives of this book is to give more detailed assistance of this type. It describes the principal tools concerned with the indexing and abstracting of medical literature and explains how they may be put to the best use. It outlines the facilities usually found in a medical library, the catalogue, classification schemes, and other arrangements made for the assistance of users. It also mentions the most important reference works, pharmaceutical, historical and biographical sources, and gives a brief account of medical library services in Britain.

Another purpose of this book is to serve as an introduction to medical librarianship for those who intend to specialize in this branch of the profession. A programme of training for health-care librarianship leading to the Library Association charter has been drawn up by the Joint Training Subcommittee of the NHS Regional Librarians Group and the University Medical School Librarians Group (Hewlett, 1988a, 1988b; Cooke et al. , 1989).

A useful handbook, *Medical librarianship*, edited by M. Carmel (1981) has been written by and for librarians practising in the medical and health-care fields and for those who wish to learn more in these special areas. A guide to information sources and to the literature of thebiomedical specialties is provided by *Information sources in the medical sciences*, written by subject specialists and edited by L.T. Morton and S. Godbolt (3rd edn., 1984; 4th edn. in preparation.). The more extensive *Handbook of medical library practice* (4th edn., 3 vols., 1982-8), is edited by L. Darling. *Medical libraries: a user guide* (Jenkins, 1987) is intended to encourage more effective use of libraries and literature among the medical profession. It includes an account of computer searching.

Two important professional journals are *Health libraries review*, Oxford, and *Bulletin of the Medical Library Association*, Chicago, both published quarterly.

2

Today the output of medical literature is enormous and it is difficult to make an informed estimate of the number of periodicals currently covering this field (see p. 14). The *Index medicus* currently indexes the contents of nearly 3,000 carefully selected journals. Expert indexing and abstracting have made this large accumulation reasonably accessible.

Experienced library users will know that to keep abreast of medical progress it is not sufficient merely to make an occasional examination of a few of the more important journals. A systematic examination of journals, abstracting services, and indexes covering the literature on his own special interests and related subjects will be a regular routine of the research worker. The general practitioner will read the periodicals of particular interest to him, supplementing them with one or more of the abstracting journals or the current-awareness service of the Royal College of General Practitioners (see p. 27). The consultant or specialist will regularly examine the periodicals and abstracting tools covering his specialty. All may wish to supplement this with tailor-made current-awareness services provided by their librarian.

The subject fields of the medical library may include chemistry, genetics, biochemistry, microbiology, anatomy, physiology, and pharmacology, as well as general medicine, surgery, obstetrics, gynaecology, and even veterinary science. Carmel (1981) has pointed out that 'Health librarianship has its own character and tradition determined by the special characteristics of its users and the unusual structure of medical knowledge. Its users are studying, teaching, and researching at the highest intellectual levels yet seldom, even in a university context, think of themselves as academics. They are practitioners and the unique nature of their practice generates a special sense of urgency and value in every supporting activity. "At the end of all our work is a patient" (Godbolt, 1977).'

We are greatly indebted to Mrs Margaret C. Stewart for help and advice during the preparation of the chapter on audio-visual aids.

L.T.M.
D.J.W.

3

2 Finding your way around the library

One of the most important parts of a medical library is the section devoted to periodicals. These are usually kept together, the bound sets on the shelves and the unbound issues within easy access. Holdings and locations of periodicals are often to be found in some form of catalogue in this section of the library as well as being in the main catalogue. Most libraries have an up-to-date handlist of current periodicals available free of charge.

Journals may be arranged on the shelves alphabetically by title or in subject groups. In some libraries the periodicals needed for reference, such as the *Index medicus* and the abstracting journals, are shelved in the reference section or some other central place. Current and other unbound issues may be placed with the bound volumes but are more often displayed on racks until a volume is completed and ready for binding.

Dictionaries, directories, encyclopaedias, data books, pharmacopoeias and drug handbooks, atlases, and other publications intended for reference only and not allowed out of the library will be found in the reference section.

The catalogue

Library catalogues are compiled to conform with well-established rules, in order to make them as consistent as possible. One may vary slightly from another to suit the particular requirements of the library it serves, but on the whole the general arrangement is well standardized. The code usually followed is the *Anglo-American cataloguing rules (AACR2).*

The catalogue may be recorded on cards, in book form, loose-leaf, on microfiche, or in a computer. The card form is still the most common although microfiches have the advantage of saving space; multiple copies can easily be made and distributed elsewhere and they can be updated frequently. In recent years some libraries have introduced computer-generated catalogues. These may be printed out on paper or in microform, keywords, or NLM (National Library of Medicine) class-marks. The latest development is the online public access catalogue, where information in the computer is accessed directly by the reader by means of a typewriter keyboard and is shown on a visual display unit. The reader may search for a book by author, title, or subject. Like the microfiche catalogue, the computer-generated catalogue may be made available in a number of places within the building and may also be accessible from outside.

CATLINE is the National Library of Medicine's online database of its holdings of monographs and first issues of periodicals, covering works published since 1801. Subject searching of this file can be carried out by means of *Medical subject headings (MeSH*, see p. 7), textwords, keywords, or NLM class-marks. A visible index such as Kardex may be used for certain purposes, such as recording the receipt of current serials. In this system cards are shingled in shallow trays and the title is written on the bottom (projecting) edge of each card, further particulars of the entry being read by raising the overlapping card. A number of trays may be stacked in a cabinet. Movable coloured signals may be used to indicate overdue or missing issues, departmental locations, etc.

Card catalogues
There are four main types of card catalogue: (1) the author (or name) catalogue, in which entries are arranged under the name(s) of author(s), institutions, and sometimes series titles; (2) the subject catalogue, where entries are arranged under specific subject headings; (3) the dictionary catalogue, where author, subject, and certain other entries are arranged together in one alphabet; and (4) the classified catalogue, in which entries are arranged in the same subject order as the classification scheme used in the library. Periodical publications,

5

transactions of societies, etc. , will usually be listed in a separate section of the catalogue or in a visible index such as Kardex, mentioned above.

A catalogue entry will give details of author(s) or corporate bodies responsible for the publication, title, number of pages, illustrations, figures or diagrams, place of publication, publisher, and date. Sometimes an annotation will be added, providing further information. At the top of the card a classification symbol or shelf mark will indicate the location of the publication.

Alphabetical arrangement
Two methods of alphabetical arrangement are in use: word by word ('nothing before something'), and letter by letter ('solidly'). The first is more popular.

Examples:

Nothing before something	*Solidly*
New, John	New, John
New Forest	Newark
New Sydenham Society	New Forest
Newark	Newspapers
Newspapers	New Sydenham Society

Proper names beginning with M', Mac, Mc, St, Ste, are arranged as if spelt Mac, Saint, Sainte. Personal and proper names containing apostrophes (O'Connor, O'Rourke, etc.) are arranged as if one word. The *Anglo-American cataloguing rules* give authoritative rulings on the form of arrangement of authors' names.

Except in geographical names and surnames, definite and indefinite articles are ignored in alphabetical arrangement. Geographical names vary: El Salvador, but Hague, The.

The German modified vowels ä, ö, ü, are usually treated as if spelt ae, oe, ue. Characters such as å, ö, ñ, ø, in Scandinavian and other languages are arranged as if a, n, o, because they are not modified letters but additional letters of their alphabets and are (with the exception of ñ) arranged after the letter z in their respective dictionaries, an arrangement that would cause confusion if followed outside their countries.

Computer catalogues

Computer-produced catalogues are essentially databases, with retrieval on certain specified fields. For example, the names of authors, subjects, titles, publishers and dates would be placed in retrieval fields, but the collation is usually placed in a non-retrieval field. The process for retrieval varies from system to system, but is usually via a menu:

A   search by personal author
B   search by corporate author
C   search by subject
D   search by title
E   search by date
F   search by ISBN

In the above example, pressing one of the keys A-F would usually prompt the searcher for the sequence of letters or numbers to be searched for. After entering the search and pressing the return key, the system will usually tell how many records contain the search key and will ask the searcher to press another key to display them on the screen or print them out on the printer. Searches can usually be made on very specific topics by the use of Boolean logic (see the section on literature searching, p. 34). The records in a computer system are filed in random order within the system, but it is essential to ensure that search terms (i.e. names of authors, subjects, etc. are entered correctly or the result will be nil. Some systems have a facility to enable the searcher to browse among similarly spelt, or adjacent, terms.

Subject headings
The subject headings in a catalogue are usually based on an accepted standard list of terms. *Medical subject headings (MeSH)*, compiled by the National Library of Medicine for use in the *Index medicus* and elsewhere, may be used for this purpose. It is revised annually and is published as Part 2 of the January issue of the Index and is also included in the annual *Cumulated index medicus* (see p. 25). It may need some modification of spelling to conform with British usage (e.g. *oesophagus* for *esophagus*) and the substitution of some British terms for American equivalents (e.g. *adrenaline* for *epinephrine*) but otherwise *MeSH* provides a first-class ready-

7

made subject headings list. It includes cross references from synonymous and alternative terms. If a home-made list of subject headings is used, the librarian will need to build up a subject headings authority list, either on cards or on a computer database to ensure consistency and provide a guide to terms used in the catalogue.

Classification schemes

Classification schemes for books may be either general schemes planned to cover the whole field of knowledge or schemes devised primarily for special subject collections. As the greater part of the stock of a medical library has to deal with disease in all its aspects, schemes catering specially for medicine have often been based on schemes for the classification of disease.

Most medical libraries classify their material in accordance with one of the recognized schemes, although in some cases individual systems have been devised to suit the special needs of a particular library. An analysis of the entries in the *Directory of medical and health care libraries in the United Kingdom and the Republic of Ireland* (6th edn. , Linton, 1986) yielded the following information on the use of classification schemes in 604 British medical libraries:

National Library of Medicine	214
Dewey decimal	96
Universal decimal	45
Barnard	33
Library of Congress	26
Bliss	15
Various other named schemes	42
'Own scheme'	79
Not given or inappropriate	54

The description of some of the more important schemes which follows is necessarily brief and intended to give only an idea of the scope, notation, advantages and disadvantages of the schemes. For a more detailed account of individual systems see *A modern outline of library classification* (Mills, 1960).

National Library of Medicine classification
Apart from the Barnard classification, the National Library of Medicine classification is the only published classification scheme designed specifically for a medical collection. It is a development of the Library of Congress classification, the only difference being that it allows for specific entry, thus bringing together in one place all aspects of a topic. The notation is mixed (a combination of letters and figures). Preclinical sciences are classed under the letters QS-QZ and clinical subjects under the letter W, both undeveloped in the Library of Congress scheme.

Example:
WB   Practice of medicine
WG   Cardiovascular system
WG 200   Heart, general works
WG 201   Anatomy, histology, embryology
WG 202   Physiology. Mechanism of heart beat
WG 205   Cardiac emergencies
WG 220   Congenital heart disease

QS (Anatomy, histology, embryology) and QT (Physiology) are for the general aspects of the subjects only; material on the anatomy or physiology of a specific organ, region or system is placed in W to achieve the aim of specific entry. The notation of the Library of Congress scheme is used to classify books outside the fields of preclinical sciences and clinical medicine. During recent years more and more medical libraries have adopted the scheme, as it is updated through the annual volumes of the *Current catalog* of the National Library of Medicine (i.e. current books may be assigned numbers which are additions to the printed version of the classification.

National Library of Medicine classification, 4th edn., Washington, Govt. Printing Office, 1978, revised 1981.

Dewey decimal classification
This is a general scheme covering the whole field of knowledge. There are ten main classes numbered 0 to 9. Further subdivision is made by adding figures to the right of the main number, giving decimal subdivision; a full point is added after the third figure. The notation is numerical. The scheme is favoured by

public libraries; it allows indefinite expansion within each subject field and it is easy to follow. A disadvantage is that it widely separates literature dealing with the various aspects of an organ, region or system.

Example:

6	Useful arts
61	Medicine
611	Anatomy
611.1	Cardiovascular system
612	Physiology
612.1	Cardiovascular system
616	Internal and clinical medicine
616.1	Cardiovascular system
616.12	Heart disease

The subdivisions . 1 to . 8 are the same for Anatomy (611), Physiology (612) and Clinical medicine (616). Auxiliary tables permit indication of form, language, time, etc. where these are required.

Dewey decimal classification and relative index, 20th edn. , 4 vols. , Albany, N.Y., Forest Press, 1989.

Universal decimal classification

This is an expansion of the Dewey decimal classification and the main classes and subdivisions correspond with those of Dewey. It is particularly useful for large collections or where very detailed classification is necessary. Its advantages and disadvantages are similar to those of Dewey; an additional criticism is that its numbers may be very long and unwieldy.

BS1000M Universal decimal classification. International medium edition. Part 1, Systemic tables; Part 2, Alphabetical index, London, British Standards Institution, 1985-8.

Barnard classification

This scheme was devised by the late C.C. Barnard in 1936 for his own library at the London School of Hygiene and Tropical Medicine. In 1955 he revised the scheme to make it more useful for all types of medical libraries. The scheme's underlying principle is that of specific entry – one place for each topic,

where all its aspects are grouped. The notation is alphabetical: there are 26 main classes, designated by the letters of the alphabet. Auxiliary tables provide for general and special needs.
Example:

O	Cardiology
OA	Blood pressure
OB	Hypertension
OOJ	Heart failure
OOJ.RRV	Catheterization of the heart

.RRV is an auxiliary subdivision used to indicate catheterization or intubation whenever it is necessary to do so. Besidesthe London School of Hygiene, the scheme is in use at the National Institute for Medical Research and elsewhere.

Barnard, C.C. *A classification for medical andveterinary libraries*, 2nd edn. , London, H.K. Lewis,1955.

Library of Congress scheme
This general scheme, devised specially for the Library of Congress, Washington, is most suitable for very large collections such as university libraries. A mixed notation is used. The various fields of knowledge are indicated by letters of the alphabet, with a second letter to indicate the principal subdivisions of each field. Further subdivision is by the use of figures. Class Q covers science, including preclinical medical subjects and Class R is devoted to medicine.
Example:

R	Medicine (general)
RC	Internal medicine. Practice of medicine
RC 666-701	Disease of the circulatory (cardio-vascular) system
RC 681-687	Diseases of the heart
RC 685	Individual diseases of the heart, A-Z
RC 685.A6	Angina pectoris

This is an excellent scheme for general libraries although it does not bring together all aspects of information on organs, systems, or regions of the body, but widely separates them.

Library of Congress classification. Class R, Medicine, 5th edn. , Washington DC, Library of Congress, 1986.

Bliss classification

This very detailed scheme is designed to encompass all branches of knowledge. It is not surprising, therefore, that it was chosen for use in the library of the Department of Health and Social Security, the Institute of Psychiatry library, and some other medical libraries. It was first published in 1940-53; a second edition, revised by the Bliss Classification Association, is in course of publication in 20 volumes. It has an alphabetical notation and is a faceted scheme, with many different arrangements possible. Class H of the second edition was published in 1980 and includes anthropology, human biology, and health sciences. The preferred citation order is 1 Person; 2 Part, organ or system; 3 Process; 4 Action; 5 Agent (following the principle of general before specific), but allowance is made for alternative citation orders.

Example:

HWE	Respiratory system	
HWF	Pharynx	
HWFT	Tonsils	
HWFT GL		Surgery
HWFT GNG		Tonsillectomy
HWG	Larynx	
HWG GL	Surgery	
HWG GNG		Laryngectomy

Mills, J. & Broughton, V. *Bliss bibliographic classification. Class H: Anthropology, human biology, health sciences*, 2nd edn. , London, Butterworths,1980.

12

3 Periodicals

A periodical (or serial) publication may be defined as a publication issued in successive parts at regular or irregular intervals and intended to be continued indefinitely. Such works as annual reviews, the *Advances* series (Academic Press and Year Book Publishers) and the proceedings and transactions of societies are usually classified as periodicals. The transactions and proceedings of congresses are not periodicals.

Periodicals form the major part of the contents of a live medical library, whose status may be assessed by its holdings of current serials rather than by the number of textbooks and monographs it possesses. In a library serving consultants, specialists, research workers and hospital staff, subscriptions to periodicals and the cost of binding them will account for the major part of its annual budget.

Origin and development

Scientific and medical journals first made their appearance in the latter half of the seventeenth century, either as the transactions of learned societies, reproducing the texts of papers delivered at their meetings, or as journals published by individuals and societies and containing papers from a variety of sources.

As early general scientific journals were followed by others devoted to special branches of science, so the general medical journals were followed by others specializing in particular branches of medicine. Today specialization is almost the rule among new journals and, as well as broad specialization in such fields as biochemistry, there are extremely specialized journals covering, for example, reconstructive microsurgery and cranio-facial genetics. Kronick (1976) has made an extensive study of the origin and development of scientific periodicals, including medical titles, from 1665 to 1790, and Porter (1964) has written an interesting paper on the history of the scientific journal, on the occasion of the 300th anniversary of the *Philosophical transactions of the Royal Society of London*.

It is difficult to determine the number of biomedical periodicals current today. In 1912 it was estimated at 1654; in 1973 Howard-Jones provided evidence that, including journals considered indispensible to medical science, such as *Nature* and *Science*, it was about 7,000, and that since 1880 the number has doubled every 33 years, implying that today there are over 8,000. However, the *Index medicus* indexes fewer than 3,000. In calculating the rate of growth of scientific periodical literature account must also be taken of increases in the thickness of volumes. Orr and Leeds (1964) found that during the period 1941-61 the average thickness of a fairly large sample of scientific journals increased by 28%: a doubling time of over 60 years. They also estimated the net growth in the number of biomedical periodicals during 1950-60 as 7%, a doubling time of 100 years. Combining the two doubling times they calculated that the growth rate during the 1950s indicated a doubling time of 38 years. However, Dannatt and Liepa (1981), after examining statistics of growth in size and numbers in the 1970s, suggested that the new biomedical literature is not expanding but contracting. See also Morton (1990).

Types

Fox (1965), a former editor of the *Lancet*, divided journals into two types – recorders and newspapers. Recorders, he wrote, are intended for the expert, giving him a means of informing his fellow experts of his investigations and experiments. The *Biochemical Journal* and the *Journal of experimental medicine* are periodicals of this type. The newspaper type, wrote Fox, is intended for the reader rather than the contributor, helping to promote the application of comparison and contact. General medical journals such as the *Lancet*, the *British medical journal*, and the *New England journal of medicine* are both recorders and newspapers.

Howard-Jones (1973) classified journals into three categories – primary, secondary and tertiary. Primary journals are those reporting first-hand observations made in the clinic, the laboratory, or in the field; specialist journals may be included in this category. Dannatt (1984) has published a detailed survey of primary sources of medical information. Secondary journals are those intended to indicate what has been published in the primary journals; they are the abstracting journals and the indexes, e.g. the *Excerpta medica* series and the *Index medicus*. Tertiary journals neither record original observations nor simply list or abstract them; they review present knowledge on a particular subject by reference to the relevant literature (e.g. *Annual review of biochemistry*). The preparation of such reviews may involve reference first to secondary literature to find out what has been written on the subject in the primary journals.

Dannatt and Liepa (1981), on the other hand, divide periodicals into two main types – primary, including recorders, newspapers and reviews, and secondary, such as the *Index medicus* and *Current contents*, which provide access to the primary types.

Lists of periodicals

Garrison (1934) compiled a chronological list of the medical and scientific periodicals published in the seventeenth and eighteenth centuries. In it he included ten medical journals appearing in the seventeenth century and 422 in the eighteenth (although some of the titles listed cannot really be regarded as periodicals). The eighteenth-century medical journals are classified by subject and divided by decade. Kronick (1958) published a list of addenda and corrigenda to Garrison's list which added a further 192 items.

Another chronological list, covering medical periodicals issued in all British territories from the seventeenth century to 1938 was compiled by LeFanu (1938). A revised edition of the list up to 1899 was published in 1984, containing 883 additions, including four published before 1684, the starting date of the original edition. Over 1,300 titles are included, with location in a few selected libraries. As far as Great Britain and Ireland are concerned, the list was extended to 1961 by Shadrake (1963), and these two lists may be complemented by *British medical*

15

periodicals, the last edition of which was published by the British Council in 1980.

Biomedical serials 1950-1960 is a selective list of periodicals in the National Library of Medicine (Spanier, 1962). There are 8939 titles in the list, which comprises periodicals current at some time between 1950 and 1960. Entry information includes title, publishing or issuing body, place of publication, volumes and dates of holdings in the library, frequency of publication and notes of title changes, summaries provided, cumulated indexes, etc. This list is particularly useful because it gives volumes and dates of sets; another useful feature is its cross references from the English translation of Japanese titles (so often used in citations in the western world) to the transliterated originals.

Biomedical serials 1950-1960 is in direct line of succession to alphabetical lists of titles of medical periodicals indexed in the *Index-catalogue of the Library of the Surgeon General's Office*. These appeared in volume 16 of the first series of the *Index-catalogue*, 1895, with a second list (including journals current in 1895) published at the conclusion of the second series in 1916 and supplements in succeeding volumes. These lists are helpful in tracing and verifying titles of older or lesser-known journals.

The most up-to-date list of important biomedical journals is that listing the journals indexed in *Index medicus*. It is revised each year and published in the January issue of the *Index* and also in the annual *Cumulated index medicus*. It is in two sections – an alphabetical listing by abbreviated titles followed by full title, and an alphabetical listing by full title followed by abbreviated title. The list is also published separately (annually) as *List of journals indexed in Index medicus* and this contains two additional sections – alphabetical listings by subject and by country. Since 1985 the style of abbreviation of titles has conformed to the rules of the *American National Standard for Information Sciences: National standard for the abbreviation of titles of publications ANSI Z39,5* 1985. In 1989 the *Index medicus* list contained 2,888 titles.

Excerpta Medica, the comprehensive abstracting service, publishes annually a *List of journals abstracted* in its publications, with full and abbreviated forms of each title. About 3,500 titles are listed.

The BioSciences Information Service (BIOSIS) of *Biological abstracts* publishes an annual list of those periodicals from which it selects and abstracts papers.

World medical periodicals, 3rd edn., World Medical Association, 1961, with supplement 1968, is an alphabetical listing of 4,732 current medical, dental, pharmaceutical and veterinary journals, together with 1,074 items which ceased to be current in recent years. It includes an index of the principal abstracting journals. Information given includes subject and country indexes.

Ulrich's international periodicals directory, published annually (28th edn., New York, Bowker, 1989-90) lists over 111,600 titles of periodicals currently in print, arranged under broad subject headings and with an alphabetical title index. It is supplemented by *Ulrich's quarterly*.

Swets serials catalogue, an annual published by Swets and Zeitlinger, Lisse, Netherlands, and supplied to its subscription customers, lists about 30,000 titles, including serials on compact disk.

The *World list of scientific periodicals*, 4th edn., 3 vols., London, 1963-5, includes periodicals current at any time between 1900 and 1960 and indicates their location in nearly 300 libraries in Britain. It lists about 60,000 titles, including medical journals, and includes proceedings of international congresses. Another important source for the location of periodicals in Britain is the *British union-catalogue of periodicals (BUCOP)* which 'provides a record of periodicals of the world from the seventeenth century to the present day, in British libraries'. It appeared in four volumes in 1955-8 with a supplement in 1962, and in fact covers the literature to 1960. In 1964 the National Central Library, now absorbed in the British Library, assumed responsibility for its continuation (incorporating the *World list*) by publishing a quarterly list of new periodicals cumulated into an annual volume. *New periodical titles 1960-68* was published in 1970 to cumulate the first five of these volumes, and a second cumulation (1969-73) appeared in 1976. *New periodical titles* ceased publication after the 1980 volume. It was succeeded by *Serials in the British Library*, 1981- , a quarterly listing with annual cumulation, which gives title, place of publication, publisher, date of commencement, and frequency. It is published by the British National Bibliographic Service, British Library, London. It includes new periodicals taken by a number of British libraries, with locations. A microfiche cumulation covering 1976-86 (57,000 titles) is also available.

In recent years the British Library Document Supply Centre (see p. 76), with its fast and efficient service, has been the main source of supply of loans and photocopies for libraries. However, now that the British Library Board has decided that the service must be realistically priced, many libraries are looking to other sources of supply. Although the *World list* and *BUCOP* are out of date they are still of use in tracing the location of older literature.

A useful list is D.P. Woodworth and C. Goodair's *Current British periodicals, 5th edn*, published by the BLDSC and UK Serials Group, 1989. This edition has about 8,600 entries, including over 4,400 amendments and 1700 new titles.

In the UK some regional librarians have compiled union-lists of the journals in the medical libraries within their Regions, and have even included selective holdings of major libraries outside their sphere of influence. The union-lists of the East Anglian and North-East Thames Regions, for example, both include selective holdings of the British Medical Association Library.

Journals in translation is a joint publication of the British Library Document Supply Centre and the International Translations Centre, Delft. It lists over 1,000 foreign journals available in cover-to-cover translation into English and has a keyword-in-context subject index.

Selection of periodicals

Numerous attempts have been made to assess the relative value of medical periodicals. Such assessments may be useful to librarians with small budgets or to readers wishing to examine only a few journals regularly. Various indicators adopted as measures – citation counts, library borrowing statistics, examination of the 'best' periodicals in a given field, etc. – have been critically examined by Dannatt (1984). The *Abridged index medicus* (1970-) indexes papers from 118 carefully selected English-language periodicals but this publication is heavily biased (75%) in favour of American publications. 'Selected list of books and journals for the small medical library' (Brandon and Hill, 1989) also has a strong American bias. It is revised about every two years. A select list, *Books and periodicals for medical libraries in hospitals*, was published by the Medical Section of the Library Association, the fifth and last edition appearing in 1978.

Guidance on the periodicals most suitable to a specialist medical library may be obtained by examination of abstracting journals devoted to the specialty or from the specialist chapters in Morton and Godbolt (1984).

4   Indexes and abstracts

Indexes

Surgeon General's catalogue

We are indebted to the United States of America for some of the most important indexes to medical literature. The Surgeon General's Library, later renamed the Armed Forces Medical Library and since 1956 known as the National Library of Medicine, is located at Bethesda, near Washington, and forms an integral part of the National Institutes of Health. It is probably the largest medical library in the world, with immense collections of books, journals, pamphlets, photographs, etc. relating to aspects of medicine and related disciplines.

The books and pamphlets, together with most of the papers in the periodical medical literature, were formerly indexed in the *Index-catalogue of the Library of the Surgeon General's Office*, providing the most exhaustive bibliography of world medical literature. The *Index-catalogue* was conceived by John Shaw Billings (1838-1913), a distinguished American librarian. Billings was given the responsibility of developing the Surgeon General's Library and set out to build up an extensive collection and to prepare a comprehensive catalogue of it. In 1876 he circulated a *Specimen fasciculus of a catalogue of the National Medical Library*, an author and subject catalogue in dictionary form, very similar to the *Index-catalogue* as it eventually appeared.

The *Specimen fasciculus* was well received and Billings proceeded with the compilation of the *Index-catalogue*. The first volume appeared in 1880 and publication proceeded at the rate of a volume a year, each volume covering one or more letters of the alphabet. On completion of the alphabet a new series was begun, again working through the alphabet and indexing literature that had accumulated in the interim. Publication in this form ceased in the middle of the fourth series owing to the inability of the *Index-catalogue* to cope with the rapid increase in volume of medical literature. The alphabetical arrangement of the *Index-catalogue* led to large accumulations of material that might wait as long as 20 years before appearing in it (see Rogers and Adams, 1950, for an account of its history). The volumes available are:

1st series: Vol. 1-16   1880-95
2nd series: Vol. 1-21   1896-1916
3rd series: Vol. 1-10   1918-32
4th series: Vol. 1-11 (A-Mn)   1936-55

A fifth series containing selected monographic material appeared in three volumes, 1959-61, the first containing author entries and the other two subject entries. These 61 volumes record 540,000 books and 2,556,000 journal articles.

To supplement the *Index-catalogue* there are:

Armed Forces Medical Library catalog 1950-1954, 6 vols. 1955
National Library of Medicine catalog 1955-1959, 6 vols. 1960
National Library of Medicine catalog 1960-1965, 6 vols. 1966
National Library of Medicine current catalog 1966- (see below)

In the first four series of the *Index-catalogue* it is possible to find entries for almost every published item of medical interest from the introduction of printing to the mid-twentieth century. Books, pamphlets, theses, etc. are entered under both author and subject; papers published in journals are indexed by subject only. The *Index-catalogue* and its successors of course deal only with material actually in the Surgeon General's Library (National Library of Medicine) although they are so comprehensive that many users have come to regard them as providing a complete bibliography of medical literature. The earlier volumes of the first series, however, were compiled

21

when the Library lacked many of the older books and it is sometimes necessary to consult the later series to find books published many years earlier. Besides this, Billings was a little selective in indexing articles from periodicals.

In 1926 a change of policy resulted in the omission of subject entries for material published after 1925, a policy fortunately reversed in 1932; users of the catalogue must therefore remember that a gap exists in the *subject* entries of books and periodicals published during the period 1926-32, involving the letters Ge-Z in the third series; this gap was partly filled in the fourth series. To cover the gap it is necessary to consult the *Index medicus* and the *Quarterly cumulative index medicus* (described below).

National Library of Medicine current catalog

January 1966 saw the appearance of the *National Library of Medicine current catalog*, published twice a month with quarterly and annual cumulations. The *Catalog* now appears quarterly, with annual cumulation. There have been two larger cumulations. In the first (for 1966-70, 7 vols.) one retrospective year (1965), which had been converted to machine-readable form, was added in order to present a comprehensive listing of cataloguing data in this form. In the second cumulation (1971-5, 5 vols.) the fifth volume is devoted to serials and is divided into subject and name sections.

Each medical title in the *Catalog* contains a classification notation according to the *National Library of Medicine classification*. Where possible, full names and dates of authors are given.

The National Library of Medicine has made available weekly sets of proof sheets of the *Catalog*, with monthly indexes, a particularly useful service for libraries using it for cataloguing purposes. These sheets may be purchased from the Medical Library Association, 6 North Michigan Avenue, Suite 300, Chicago, Ill. 60602, USA. This cataloguing information is also available from NLM on CATLINE (see p. 5).

Index medicus 1879-1927

The *Index medicus* was launched in 1879 by John Shaw Billings with the assistance of Robert Fletcher, who qualified in medicine in Bristol and emigrated to the USA. It first appeared monthly, was suspended in April 1899, and resumed publication in 1903. It has a classified subject arrangement. Each volume was provided with separate author and subject indexes until 1920, after which it contained only author indexes. It indexed about half the current journals listed in the *Index-catalogue* and included some books. The gap 1899-1902 is rather inadequately filled by *Bibliographia medica* (3 vols., Paris, 1900-3) and *Index medicus novus* (Vienna, 1899-1900).

In 1916 the American Medical Association began publication of the *Quarterly cumulative index to current medical literature*, which in 1927 was amalgamated with the *Index medicus* to form the *Quarterly cumulative index medicus*.

Quarterly cumulative index medicus

This was a co-operative production of the American Medical Association and the Surgeon General's Library until 1931, when the AMA assumed sole responsibility for it. Each volume has, in one alphabetical sequence, author and subject entries for papers published in about 1,400 journals, and, in a separate section, similar entries for new books. Until 1940 the *QCIM* appeared quarterly, the first and third quarters being cumulated into the second and fourth, providing two permanent volumes for each year (January-June and July-December). A list of the journals indexed in each volume is included, together with the names and addresses of book publishers.

Like similar indexes, the *QCIM* could never be quite up to date; if a reference cannot be found in the issues for the appropriate year, issues for the next year at least should be consulted. During the 1939-45 war, European literature reached the USA either very late or not at all, and users of the *QCIM* must bear in mind that many papers published during this period may be indexed several years late or may not be found at all.

Even in normal times the inevitable delay between publication of a paper and its appearance in the *QCIM* was an inconvenience to those seeking the most recent literature. Delay in publication during the war was followed by post-war production difficulties and eventually volumes were appearing more than two years late. Fortunately by this time a reasonable and up-to-date alternative, the *Current list of medical litera-ture* had become well established and by the time the 1956 volumes of the *QCIM* appeared plans were already in hand for a new *Index medicus*.

Current list of medical literature

During the 1939-45 war a more rapid indexing service than that provided by the *Quarterly cumulative index medicus* was essential. This was provided by the *Current list of medical literature*, which first appeared in 1941 as a pocket-size index, to be displaced in due course by the *QCIM*. It was taken over by the Armed Forces Medical Library in 1945 and from 1950 appeared monthly, with author and subject indexes and cumulated half-yearly indexes. Its value lay in the fact that papers were indexed in it within two or three months of publication. In each issue journals are arranged alphabetically by title and each entry gives author, title (with translation in the case of foreign items), and inclusive pagination. One disadvantage of the *Current list* is that an index must be consulted in order to turn to the reference sought. About a third of the journals indexed are not covered by the *QCIM*.

Index medicus 1960-

In January 1960 the *Current list* was replaced by a new *Index medicus*, issued monthly and cumulated annually to form the *Cumulated index medicus*. Each issue has three sections: the first providing a bibliography of medical reviews, the second giving subject entries to journal articles, and the third author entries. In addition, the January issue contains a list of the journals currently indexed: an alphabetical listing of the journal title abbreviation used in the *Index* followed by the full title, and an alphabetical listing by the full title followed by the abbreviated form. This list of journals is also published separately each year as *List of journals indexed in index medicus* and in this form contains two additional sections providing subject and geographical indexes. The abbreviations used for journal titles conform to the rules of the American National Standard for Information Sciences: *National stan-dard for the abbreviation of titles of periodicals, ANSI Z39. 5* 1985.

The *Index medicus* indexes some 250,000 papers a year from about 2,750 journals. The January issue is published in two parts, the second of which is entitled *Medical subject headings (MeSH)*, a list of the subject headings and cross references used in *Index medicus*.

Included in each issue of *Index medicus* is a section entitled 'Bibliography of medical reviews', a valuable source for tracing review articles, selected from journals covered for *Index medicus*. Until 1987, the NLM defined medical reviews as well-documented surveys of the recent biomedical literature but in 1988 this definition was broadened to encompass reviews of current thinking on a given subject, regardless of the age of the literature cited. A useful feature of the 'Bibliography' is that the number of references cited in each article indexed is given. The 'Bibliography' was begun as a separate publication in 1955 and there are cumulations covering 1955-60, 1966-70, 1971-5 and 1975-80. Annual cumulations are included in the *Cumulated index medicus*. *Index medicus* is available online (see p. 35).

The annual *Cumulated index medicus*, published since 1960, contains *MeSH*, the *List of journals indexed*, the 'Bibliography of medical reviews', and the cumulated subject and author indexes of references in the monthly issues.

In 1980 the National Library of Medicine began publication of the *Abridged index medicus*, with annual cumulation in *Cumulated abridged index medicus* modelled on the *Index medicus* and containing citations to 118 English-language journals. The low cost of this abridged index makes it attractive to small libraries taking comparatively few journals. It has a noticeable American bias.

The policy governing the selection of journals for inclusion in *Index medicus* is outlined in the January issue each year. This is also outlined by Karel (1967) who gives a brief historical sketch of some earlier medical bibliographies. A detailed account of the *Index medicus* from 1879 has been published by Sutherland (1984).

Current contents
A useful current-awareness tool is the *Current contents* series, which appear weekly and reproduce the contents pages of

about 6,500 journals. Three of the series are of interest to medicine: *Current contents, life sciences* (1,150 journals); *Current contents, clinical medicine* (850 journals); and *Current contents, social and behavioral sciences* (1,300 journals) which is of most interest to the psychiatrist, the psychologist, and the social worker. There is a certain amount of overlap in coverage by the three series. Each series includes the section 'Current book contents' in which book series, reviews, proceedings, etc. are selectively listed with bibliographical details. Each issue has a list of the journals appearing in it, addresses of first authors of papers listed, and a subject index. An updated list of the journals covered is published twice a year, with addresses of publishers; and a triannual journal index is also provided. The *Life sciences* and *Clinical medicine* series are also available online. *Current contents* is publishedin the USA by the Institute for Scientific Information, Philadelphia, and reaches Britain before some of the journals listed in it. It is particularly useful to the librarian for monitoring journals not taken by the library or not easily accessible first hand, and for checking references to papers published too recently to be in *Index medicus*.

Other indexes

The National Library of Medicine publishes a series of current bibliographies in medicine. Subscribers receive approximately 20 bibliographies annually, dealing with distinct subject areas. Titles of these bibliographies are to be found in each monthly issue of *Index medicus*. In addition the NLM publishes *AIDS bibliography*, a quarterly list of references to relevant books and journal articles.

Excerpta Medica Foundation and its associate Elsevier publish

Adverse reaction titles(monthly)
Clinical chemistry lookout (monthly)
Current titles and abstracts in immunology (twice a month)
Transplantation and allergy (twice a month).

The last two are a mixture of titles and abstracts.

The Oncology Information Service, based at the Medical and Dental Library, Leeds University, publishes 22 monthly current-awareness bulletins, each covering the literature on a specific aspect of clinical cancer. Each bulletin is a list of references retrieved by scanning 1,000 journals. The Service also publishes *AIDS information* monthly.

New reading for general practitioners, an annotated list of books and journal articles, is published by the Royal College of General Practitioners (p. 71). It is updated quarterly.

The *Index to dental literature* is produced by the National Library of Medicine and published by the American Dental Association. It indexes 1,400 journals and lists new books. It appears in four cumulations a year, the last being a hardback.

A bibliography of nursing literature 1859-1960, was compiled by Alice M.C. Thompson, London, Library Association for Royal College of Nursing, 1968. A supplement for 1961-70 in two volumes (1974) was also the work of Thompson, and two further supplements for 1971-5 and 1976-80, compiled and edited by Frances Walsh, appeared in 1985. These volumes reflect the enormous increase in the amount of nursing literature published in recent years. Both compilers were librarians of the Royal College of Nursing. Since 1972 the College has published a monthly *Nursing Bibliography*, and an index of nursing research is maintained at the Department of Health and Social Security (p. 31).

The *Hospital literature index*, published by the American Hospital Association since 1945, gives a wide coverage of the subject. It is published quarterly with annual cumulations.

The *Index-catalogue of medical and veterinary zoology*, Washington, U.S. Dept. of Agriculture, 1932- , is an exhaustive index of the literature on animal parasites of man and animals. The main body of the work is arranged alphabetically under authors, with volumes devoted to specific subjects. Besides articles in periodicals it includes references to books, congresses, theses, etc.

In recent years a method of information access using citations given in published papers has become available. Eugene Garfield, a pioneer in this field, has defined a citation index as 'an ordered list of references (cited works) in which each reference is followed by a list of the sources (citing works) which cite it' (Garfield, 1964, 1970). Its main purpose is to lead the searcher from a key paper to others which have referred to it, on the assumption that they will be relevant. It enables the user to trace new applications and improvements of theories, methods, instruments, etc. and makes it easy to locate corrections, amendments, refutations, discussions, etc. The *Science citation index* is produced by the Institute for Scientific Information, Philadelphia. It is published every two months, with annual cumulations. It first appeared in 1961 and then annually from 1964. Its components are a citation index, a corporate index, a source index, and a 'permuterm' subject index. The *Science citation index* now deals with the citations published in about 5,000 source journals. It is also available online as SCISEARCH (over 6,000,000 citations). In addition, ISI operates a personal service, ASCA (Automatic Subject Citation Alert). For each search a profile is prepared containing a number of keywords, authors' names, etc. and once a week a print-out containing matching references is mailed to the customer. A guide, 'How to use the Science Citation Index', by E. Garfield, appears in the SCI Guide each year.

Book lists

Mention has already been made of the *National Library of Medicine current catalog* (p. 22). The *Cumulative book index*, published monthly except in August and later cumulated, indexes all English-language books by author, title and subject. The *British national bibliography* appears weekly but is confined to books published in Britain.

Books in print (New York, Bowker), published annually, with a mid-year supplement, gives a complete listing of American books in print, arranged by author, title, and subject.

British books in print (London, Whitaker). the British equivalent of Bowker's *Books in print*, provides an annual listing of books published in Britain.

Bowker's *Medical and health care books and serials in print*, published annually, gives bibliographical details of textbooks, monographs, reference works, etc. published in the USA, British books which have American publishers, and serials published throughout the world. There are three sections for books, which are listed by subject, author and title. The serials index comprises about 9000 entries, under both subjects and titles.

28

British medicine, published monthly by Pergamon Press, with the support of the Royal Society of Medicine, lists new books, non-book material, research reports, official publications, etc. originating in the British Commonwealth.

Extensive lists of books on general medicine and its specialties are to be found in most chapters of *Information sources in the medical sciences* (Morton and Godbolt, 1984).

Books at Boston Spa is a microfiche listing of all Western European-language monographs published since 1980 that are held at the British Library Document Supply Centre at Boston Spa. These number over 280,000.

CATLINE, the National Library of Medicine's online database of monographs and first issues of periodicals, covers works published since 1801. Subject searching of CATLINE can be carried out by means of *MeSH* headings, textwords, keywords, or NLM class-marks.

Theses and dissertations

The *British theses service (BRITS), an index to the British thesis collections (1971-1987) held at the British Library Document Supply Centre and London University* is published by IPI Limited, Godstone, Surrey, 1989, in three volumes. There is to be an annual update.

A guide to British theses, listed by subject with an author index, is provided by Aslib's *Index to theses accepted for higher degrees by the universities of Great Britain and Ireland and the Council for National Academic Awards* (1950/51-). This appears twice a year and lists about 9,000 theses a year. *Dissertation abstracts international* lists and abstracts North American doctoral theses and some from European universities. It is published by University Microfilm International, Ann Arbor, Michigan. Theses listed are also available on microfilm and on CD-ROM. *British reports, translations and theses* is published monthly by the British Document Supply Centre with annual cumulations. A keyterm index is included in each part. Author, report number and keyterm indexes are provided on microfiche in the March, June, September and December issues.

A copy of all theses accepted for higher degrees is deposited in the library of the university, medical school or medical faculty concerned and may be available for consultation or on inter-library loan. For further information on theses see Dannatt (1984).

Abstracting services

Today it is not possible for a medical scientist or a specialist to read everything being published within his field of interest. He must utilize abstracting services as well as current journals and current-awareness services.

Only the principal abstracting services can be mentioned here; more extensive guides have been published by Roper and Boorkman (1980), and by Dalby (1975) (which includes current-awareness services). *Ulrich's international periodicals directory* (New York, Bowker) has a comprehensive list of abstracting journals, listed under broad subject headings.

Abstracts may be divided into two types – informative and indicative. An informative abstract gives the essential details of a paper and provides all the basic information supplied by the original author, making it unnecessary for the reader to consult the original except for details of techniques, methods, case records, etc. An indicative abstract is one that merely outlines the scope of a paper, helping the reader to decide whether or not it is worth while to read the original.

An abstracting journal may provide complete coverage of the literature within its scope or it may be selective. A selective service is likely to provide critical and discursive abstracts. It will appeal particularly to those who do not wish to examine abstracts of everything published on the subject in which they are interested but are prepared to be guided by an expert who can select the most important papers.

Almost as soon as periodical literature appeared in the seventeenth century, there were attempts at digests and abstracts, and by the early part of the twentieth century medical abstracting journals had become well established. In Germany the firm of Julius Springer published a series of *Berichte* and *Zentralblätter* covering most branches of medicine and surgery. Unfortunately these journals slowly wasted away during the 1939-45 war as the periodicals on which they depended ceased to reach Germany. By 1944 they had stopped altogether. Publication of some Springer journals was resumed

30

a few years after the war and today 11 Springer titles are available.

At the end of the war the Dutch Excerpta Medica Foundation was established, one of its principal objectives being to provide a complete-cover abstracting service. It began in 1947 and today publishes 45 specialist abstracting journals covering all branches of medicine, surgery and fringe subjects and seven 'core' journals containing abstracts from top journals in various specialties. Frequency of publication of individual abstracting journals varies from 6 to 32 issues a year. Author and subject indexes are provided in each issue and are cumulated for each volume. Excerpta also publishes a range of user manuals and the annual *List of journals abstracted*. Excerpta Medica abstracting journals are also available online (EMBASE, see p. 38). EMTREE is the classification system used for this database.

The Department of Health and Social Security Library, London, publishes several monthly abstracting journals – all produced from DHSS-data, its computerized database. *Health service abstracts*, originally called *Current literature on health services*, was started in 1972 and was given its present name in 1985. It is published monthly and contains abstracts of new books, reports, and journal articles connected with the management and administration of the National Health Service. Volumes run from May to April. *Social service abstracts*, also monthly, covers the whole range of the personal social services, with particular emphasis on literature originating in Britain. *Health buildings library bulletin* is a monthly list of abstracts on the planning, design, construction and maintenance of all types of health buildings. *Nursing research abstracts* is a quarterly, based on data in the Index of nursing research and consists of details of current and published research in the UK, of relevance to nursing, midwifery and health visiting.

ASSIA – Applied social sciences index and abstracts, published every two months since 1987 by the Library Association, London, contains indicative abstracts covering a wide field that includes social medicine. It monitors 500 English-language journals. Each issue includes a subject index.

In France the Centre Nationale de la Recherche Scientifique publishes 22 bibliographies in the biomedical field. These

31

appear ten times a year. The Centre's PASCAL databases (available through DIALOG) give online access and retrospective search facilities back to 1973 and now contain 7,000,000 references. More than 8,500 scientific, technical, and medical journals are analysed.

In the USSR the *Medicinskij referativnyi zhurnal* series comprises 22 abstracting journals, each appearing monthly.

The C.A.B. International (formerly the Commonwealth Agricultural Bureaux) is responsible through associated institutes for the publication of several abstracting journals. Those of interest to medical scientists are *Helminthological abstracts, Nutrition abstracts and reviews, Review of applied entomology, Review of medical and veterinary mycology*, and the *Veterinary bulletin*.

In the field of public health and hygiene the Bureau of Hygiene and Tropical Diseases, London, publishes monthly *Abstracts on hygiene*.

Cambridge Science Abstracts, Bethesda, Md, publishes about 30 abstracting journals, of which 14 are concerned with biomedicine and most of which appear monthly. These are also available online. They also produce biomedical research databases in Compact Disk – Read-Only Memory (CD-ROM) format, including MEDLINE and CANCERLIT.

Other useful specialist abstracting journals that may be mentioned are *Ophthalmic literature*, London, 1947- , published seven times a year, containing informative abstracts, advance book reviews, an author index in each issue and annual author and subject indexes; and *Dental abstracts*, which has appeared monthly since 1956 from the American Dental Association, Chicago.

Three valuable abstracting journals of interest in the field of medical science are *Chemical abstracts, Biological abstracts*, and *Psychological abstracts*. Today the literature being published in the first field is so prolific that *Chemical abstracts* now appears weekly. Some 8,000 journals are examined for abstracting purposes and 600,000 abstracts are published a year. About a third of its contents is of biochemical interest; it also deals with patent literature. It has good author and subject indexes, cumulated annually and quinquennially, and has been available online as CA SEARCH since 1967. *Biological abstracts* publishes abstracts of papers from about 8,000 journals; subjects covered include genetics, cytochemistry, biochemistry, biophysics, nutrition, physiology, experimental and clinical medicine, to name only a few. This is also available online. *Psychological abstracts* (1927-) appears monthly from Washington. It has a classified arrangement; author and subject indexes are provided in each issue and are cumulated annually. It is available online.

5 Searching the literature

Literature searches may be carried out manually or by automated means, using the many databases available.

Manual searching

For over a hundred years manual searching has been simplified by the availability of indexing and abstracting tools. The *Index medicus* (p. 24) and the *Index-catalogue* (p. 20) provide exhaustive indexes to biomedical literature. To make a complete search for literature on a given subject it would be necessary to work through the four series of the *Index-catalogue* and the subsequent volumes of the *Index medicus*. In practice it is better to work backwards from the present, bearing in mind that a good review article or book may be found that will provide references to important work published previously.

When using the *Index medicus* it is important first to check in *MeSH (Medical subject headings)* to ensure that the term used in *Index medicus* is being consulted. This is an American publication using American terms and spellings and the unfamiliar user, not finding any papers under the term being consulted, may think that nothing has been published on the topic. For example, *oestrogen* will be listed as *estrogen* and *adrenaline* will not be found at all because *epinephrine* is the term used for it in the USA. Adequate and helpful cross references are included in *MeSH*.

Under each subject heading and subheading in *Index medicus* English-language papers are arranged alphabetically by the title of the journal concerned, followed by foreign-language papers arranged alphabetically by language and cited with an English translation of the title.

When consulting *Index medicus* it is well to bear in mind the 'Bibliography of Medical Reviews' (p. 25) as a short cut to more extensive well-documented papers. Entries in the 'Bibliography' are of course repeated in the main body of *Index medicus*.

The next source for manual searching is the abstracting journal. *Excerpta medica, Chemical abstracts* and *Biological abstracts* have already been described (p. 31-2). While *Index medicus* gives only the bibliographic details of an article, an abstracting journal gives a summary or abstract of the article as well. Abstracts may help the reader to decide between papers that should be read in the original and those that should be discarded. If the original is in a foreign language an abstract may avoid the necessity of a translation. On the other hand, *Index medicus* entries appear only a few months after the publication of the original paper, whereas abstracts may appear as much as 12 months or more later.

The most important biomedical abstracting journals are the series published by the Excerpta Medica Foundation (p. 31). They cover all medical and surgical specialties. Each issue and each volume has its own author and subject indexes. Some 3,500 journals are scanned, compared with 2,750 indexed in *Index medicus*.

Computer searching

Computer databases have revolutionized literature searching. By the 1950s the publication of *Quarterly cumulative index medicus* was being seriously delayed by the cumbersome methods employed in the editorial process, especially the inter-filing of new records. The National Library of Medicine started the search for a new system to replace it, using an in-house computer. It called the new system MEDLARS (MEDical Literature Analysis and Retrieval System), and it became operational in 1960, with the publication of the new computer-produced series of *Index medicus*.

Since the NLM allowed online access to its MEDLARS database through MEDLINE (MEDlars-on-LINE) from the mid-1960s, it has been possible to supply comprehensive reference lists on almost any topic in a fraction of the time taken to search by hand.

A further major advance has been the introduction of Compact Disk – Read-Only Memory (CD-ROM). The disks are read by a CD drive attached to a microcomputer and use all the techniques of online searching without the online telecommunication costs. Each disk is five inches in diameter and can hold a complete year of MEDLINE, or a comparable amount of any other database.

A computer database is composed of records – one record for each book, journal article or other item of information. Each record is divided into fields, e.g. the author field, the title field, date field, and so on. By entering a search term and matching it against the relevant field(s) in a record, the computer will identify which records are required and will display them on the screen or print them out, as required.

For all computer searching it is probably best to spend a little time beforehand formulating your search. Most databases allow the use of free text searching (i.e. words which occur in the search statement can be entered exactly as they are), but some only permit the use of terms that are included in the thesaurus issued with that system. By selecting the terms from the thesaurus that match the topic required, it is possible to have a list of relevant references in a fraction of the time that it takes to search manually, and search terms can be combined using Boolean logic to specify the exact topic.

Boolean logic uses the operators *and*, *or*, and *not* to combine terms or to exclude terms. For example

THORACIC DISEASES AND STRESS

will find references which include both terms, and therefore are concerned with stress-induced chest diseases;

THORACIC DISEASES OR STRESS

will find references which contain either term, so therefore are not specifically on stress-induced chest diseases, but on either chest diseases or on stress;

THORACIC DISEASES NOT STRESS

will find references on chest diseases that are not stress-induced.

Compact disks

These are now standard equipment in many libraries, and are usually available for end-user searching by readers. The equipment needed is a microcomputer, software, compact disk drive and a printer (to provide hard copy of the search results). All the versions of databases on compact disk are menu-driven, so no previous experience is necessary. Most libraries will allocate a time slot (say, half an hour), and there may be a small charge for print-outs. At present all systems have disk drives in which the disk has to be inserted by hand, but the British Library, together with Next Technology, has just produced the world's first multi-drive CD-ROM jukebox, storing over 250 compact disks. This can store over 175,000 Mb of computer data – over 87,000,000 pages. It is possible to search by author(s), subject heading, keyword in title, date, and many other concepts. It is helpful to decide beforehand which terms to enter first and whether to combine them with others, as it saves computer time. At any stage you can display the results of your search so far, so that you can amend, expand, or finish your search strategy.

Each menu will give you a choice of options. For example, it may ask you to enter your search term and then ask which field to match it against. When the search is finished to your satisfaction, you have the options of displaying the result on the screen, of printing out the results, or of downloading them to a floppy disk. This can then be edited by any word processing programme.

Online searching

This is basically the same technique as above, but with a few minor differences. The equipment needed is a terminal (preferably a microcomputer), a modem (for connecting the terminal to the telephone system), and a printer (for hard copy). It is also necessary to have some communication software with the microcomputer.

The search strategy is defined in the same way, and the terms are entered in the same way. However, although the references retrieved can be displayed on the screen, or downloaded, it is more usual not to print out more than a few references whilst online, as the cost can be quite high. Printouts of lists of references are normally done offline by the database host and mailed to the user. This takes about a week.

There are advantages and disadvantages with each method. Which method is preferable is dependent on a number of factors. The three major ones (the '3 Cs') are:

1   *Cost.* The cost of the respective equipment varies, so it is not possible to say which is the most expensive system. For CD-ROMs there is an annual subscription, but once you have subscribed, any use made of it incurs no further charge. With online services, as well as the annual subscription there are telecommunication charges (e.g. to British Telecom) and each time the system is used an online charge is made by the database host. A charge is also made for offline prints.

2   *Coverage.* An online service is the most comprehensive. For example, MEDLINE is available online from 1966, which means that it is possible to search the whole period since then at one search. CD-ROMs, however, are currently limited to one year per disk, and in most systems disks are available only for the past five years. Therefore, searching over a period may involve many disk changes.

3   *Currency.* Generally speaking, the online services are more up to date. Records are added to each system daily, weekly, or monthly. CD-ROMs consist of one year's records, or have a cut-off point, with the current year having, generally, three-month updates. They could, therefore, be as much as six months out of date by the time you receive your next disk.

A minor disadvantage with the online services is that whereas the reader is usually permitted to use the CD-ROM system himself, it is almost always the case that online searches can be made only by someone experienced, usually the librarian, meaning that readers have to submit their search request and wait for the result – especially if this is being printed offline to reduce the cost.

Many other databases besides MEDLINE are of course available (see Lyon, 1989), especially for abstracting journals. Among them may be mentioned EMBASE (p. 31), for searching Excerpta Medica journals; CA SEARCH, for searching *Chemical abstracts* (p. 33); SCISEARCH, for *Science citation index* (p. 28) and CATLINE for the *NLM catalog*

(p. 29). *Current contents: life sciences* and *Current contents: clinical medicine* (p. 25) may also be searched online.

For online search facilities for audio-visual aids, see p. 67. See also Welch and King (1985).

6 Basic reference works

One of the most extensive guides to reference literature in the medical field is *Medical reference works 1679-1966*, (Blake and Roos, 1967). It lists indexes, abstracting journals, reviews, bibliographies, dictionaries, historical and biographical material, etc. It has been updated by Clark (1970), Richmond (1973-5) and later by means of a section in the annual *National Library of Medicine current catalog* under the subject heading 'Reference books, medical'. A detailed account of standard reference sources in medicine – encyclopaedias, yearbooks, handbooks, annual reviews, directories, books on nomenclature, eponyms and syndromes, data books, statistical works, and current biographical sources – has been published by Hague (1984).

A comprehensive survey has been provided by Roper and Boorkman (1980): *Introduction to reference sources in the health sciences*. Although the emphasis throughout this work is on American publications, it is nevertheless a useful compilation, particularly as references for further reading are given at the end of each chapter.

The *Oxford companion to medicine*, 2 vols., Oxford, O.U.P., 1986, contains over 7,000 entries ranging from definitions to biographies and essays on major topics.

Nomenclature, terminology, dictionaries

International Anatomical Nomenclature Committee, *Nomina anatomica*. 4th edn. Amsterdam, Excerpta Medica, 1987.
The terminology is arranged first by parts of the body and then by systems.

Donath, T., *Anatomical dictionary with nomenclatures and explanatory notes.* English edition by G.N.C. Crawford, Oxford, Pergamon Press, 1963.

Brings together the Basle, Jena, and Paris nomenclatures.

International Committee for the Preparation of the Decennial Revision of International Lists of Diseases and Causes of Death, *Manual of the international statistical classification of diseases, injuries and causes of death.* 9th revision, 2 vols., Geneva, World Health Organization, 1977-8.

Royal College of Physicians of London, *The nomenclature of disease*, 8th edn., London, HMSO, 1961.

Part 1 gives a classification of disease based on aetiology; includes a list of eponyms.

Davies, P.M., *Medical terminology in hospital practice*, 4th edn., London, Heinemann Medical, 1985.

Intended as a guide to all engaged in professions allied to medicine; in essence an elementary textbook of medicine, giving brief explanations of several thousand medical terms, including prefixes and suffixes.

Roberts, Ff., *Medical terms: their origin and construction*, 5th edn., London, Heinemann Medical, 1971.

A guide to the derivation, construction and meaning of medical terms. Lists Greek and Latin combining forms, English meaning, and examples.

Skinner, H.A., *The origin of medical terms*, 2nd edn., Baltimore, Williams and Wilkins, 1961.

Lists about 4,000 commonly used terms, with detailed explanations of origin and significance. Includes some biographical material.

Blakiston's New Gould medical dictionary, 4th edn., New York, McGraw Hill, 1979.

Comprehensive; includes biographical sketches. First compiled by G.M. Gould, 1894.

Butterworths medical dictionary, 2nd edn., London, Butterworths, 1978.

Comprehensive; includes brief biographical notes, eponyms, abbreviations. English (as opposed to American) spellings.

Churchill's illustrated medical dictionary, New York, Churchill Livingstone, 1989.
Comprehensive and up to date; American and English spellings.

Dorland's illustrated medical dictionary, 27th edn., Philadelphia, W.B. Saunders, 1988.
Comprehensive; probably the most widely used medical dictionary. An abridged version is published under the title *Pocket medical dictionary* (24th edn., 1989).

Lennox, B. & Lennox, M.E., *Heinemann medical dictionary*, London, Heinemann Medical, 1986.
Almost a 'pocket' dictionary.

Stedman's medical dictionary, 24th edn., Baltimore, Williams & Wilkins, 1982
Comprehensive standard dictionary. Includes brief biographical notes and etymological word list.

Taber, C.W., *Cyclopedic medical dictionary*, 15th edn., Philadelphia, F.A. Davis, 1985.
Encyclopaedic type of dictionary; 60,000 definitions.

Sliosberg, A., *Elsevier's medical dictionary in five languages*, 2nd edn., Amsterdam, Elsevier, 1975.
Over 35,000 terms defined in English, with indexes in French, Italian, Spanish and German.

Veillon/Nobel medical dictionary, Paris, Masson, 1977.
Lists 50,000 English medical terms, with their equivalents in French and German.

Fairpo, J.E.H. & Fairpo, C.G., *Heinemann dental dictionary*, 3rd edn., London, Heinemann Medical, 1987.

Steen, E.B., *Abbreviations in medicine and the related sciences*, 5th edn., London, Baillière, 1984.
Lists 15,000 abbreviations in current use.

Landau, S.I., (ed.-in-chief), *International dictionary of medicine and biology*, 3rd edn., 3 vols. New York, Wiley, 1986.
Over 15,000 definitions.

Eponyms

Dobson, J., *Anatomical eponyms*, 2nd edn., Edinburgh, Livingstone, 1962.
Biographical dictionary of anatomists with definitions of the structures to which their names have become attached and references to the works in which they are described.

Firkin, B.G. & Whitworth, J.A., *A dictionary of medical eponyms*, Carnforth, Parthenon, 1987.

Jablonski, S., *Dictionary of syndromes and eponymic diseases*, 2nd edn., Melbourne, Fla., Krieger, 1989.
Gives names, dates, descriptions and bibliographical references.

Magalini, S. & Scrasia. E., *Dictionary of eponymic syndromes*, 2nd edn., Philadelphia, Lippincott, 1981.
Each entry includes synonyms, symptoms, signs, pathology, treatment, prognosis, and references.

Quotations

Strauss, M.B. (ed.), *Familiar medical quotations*, Boston, Little, Brown, 1968.
Over 7,000 quotations arranged by subject; dates of birth and death are appended to names but few original sources are given.

Data books

Altman, P.L. & Dittmer, D.S., *Biology data book*, 2nd edn., 3 vols. Bethesda. Md., Federation of American Societies for Experimental Biology, 1972-4.
Contains general biological data.

Fasman, G.D. (ed.), *Handbook of biochemistry and molecular biology*, 3rd edn., 8 vols. Cleveland, Ohio,CRC Press, 1975-6.

Geigy scientific tables, 8th edn., Horsham, Geigy Pharmaceuticals, 1983-6.
Intended to provide medical practitioners and research workers with basic scientific data in a concise form.

The Merck index. An encyclopedia of chemicals and drugs, 10th edn., Rahway, N.J., Merck, 1983.
Comprehensive index of information on the chemical and physical properties, doses, and toxicities of about 10,000 compounds.

Weast, R.C. (ed.), *CRC handbook of chemistry and physics*, Boca Raton, Fla., CRC Press.
A ready-reference book of chemicals and physical data. Revised about every two years.

Dawson, R.M.C. *et al.*, *Data for biochemical research*, 3rd edn., Oxford, Clarendon Press, 1986.
Information about compounds, reagents and techniques most frequently used in biochemistry and related fields.

Directories

A few of the more important biographical sources are mentioned on p. 60. A comprehensive listing of general and specialist directories is included in Blake & Roos (1967) and supplements (see p. 40).

The world of learning, London, Europa Publications.
Annual. A guide to the educational, scientific and cultural institutions of the world: universities, colleges, academies, research institutes, libraries, museums. Arranged by country, with alphabetical index of institutions.

Commonwealth universities yearbook, 4 vols., London, Association of Commonwealth Universities.
Annual. Data on the universities of the Commonwealth, including teaching and other staff, admission requirements, affiliated colleges, etc.

World directory of medical schools, 6th edn., Geneva, World Health Organization, 1988.
Lists institutions of medical education in most countries of the world. Includes conditions of admission, curriculum, examinations, qualifications and licensure, etc.

Davies, I.J.T., Handbook of postgraduate medical education for the United Kingdom, Welwyn Garden City, Update

Books, 1980.
Clarifies ways in which postgraduate medical education is planned, organized, supplied, and monitored in the UK.

Higson, N., *Directory of British postgraduate medical qualifications*, London, Chapman & Hall, 1957.
Details postgraduate courses available and the universities and institutes offering them.

General Medical Council, *List of hospital and house officer posts in the United Kingdom which are approved or recognized for preregistration service*, London, GMC.
Published about every two years.

Hospitals and health services year book, London, Institute of Hospital Services Management.
Annual. Provides information on government departments, hospitals, regional health authorities, hospital management officials, bed and patient statistics, blood transfusion services, finance, etc.

Current research in Britain, 4 vols., Boston Spa, British Library.
Comprehensive listing of research in progress, with entries arranged by institution in broad subject categories, complemented by subject, name, and institution indexes; also available online through BLAISE. Published in three annual volumes: Physical sciences, Biological sciences, and Social sciences; and one biennial volume: Humanities.

Medical research centres, 8th edn., 2 vols., London, Butterworths, 1988.
World guide to government and independent medical research establishments.

Medical Research Council, *Handbook*, London, HMSO.
Annual. Gives details of the research activities of Council research establishments and other research sponsored by the Council.

Charities Aid Foundation, *Directory of grant-making trusts*. 10th comp., Tonbridge, Charities Aid Foundation, 1987.
Lists over 2000 charitable trusts, with information on the purposes for which they make grants. Includes medical study and research.

Grants register, London, Macmillan.
Biennial. Gives information on grants available in the
English-speaking world.

Societies

International and national societies are listed in *World of
learning* (p. 44).

Verrel, B. & Opitz, H. (eds.), *World guide to scientific
associations*, New York, K.G. Saur, 1984.
Data on over 10,000 associations and societies devoted to all
fields of research as well as medical schools and
organizations.

Henderson, G.P. & S.P.A., (eds.), *Directory of British associa-
tions and associations in Ireland*, 9th edn., Beckenham, CBD
Research, 1988.
Includes medical organizations.

Congresses and conferences

British Library, *Index to conference proceedings received*,
Boston Spa, 1964-.
Monthly. Lists proceedings received at the British Library
Document Supply Centre. Subject index to each issue and
cumulated annually. Available on BLAISE.

World list of scientific periodicals, 4th edn., London, Butter-
worth, 1965.
Includes a list of published proceedings of periodical
international congresses, with holdings in British libraries.

Bishop, W.J., *Bibliography of international congresses of
medical sciences*, Oxford, Blackwell, 1958.
Lists 363 individual congresses.

Institute for Scientific Information, *Index to scientific and
technical proceedings*, Philadelphia, Institute for Scientific
Information, 1978- .
Monthly, with semi-annual cumulations. Indexes published
proceedings, including individual papers; selective.

US Library of Congress, *World list of future international meetings. Part 1: Science, technology, agriculture, medicine.* Washington, GPO, 1959- .
Quarterly. Lists meetings for three years, with monthly interim issues noting changes.

British medicine, Oxford, Pergamon.
Monthly. Announces forthcoming congresses.

Aslib, *Forthcoming international scientific and technical conferences*, London.
Quarterly.

Council for International Organizations of Medical Sciences, *Calendar of congresses of medical sciences*, Geneva.
Annual. Lists forthcoming congresses, giving subject, place, date, and name and address of organizer.

Cambridge Scientific Abstracts, Bethesda, Md. has published *Conference papers index* every two months since 1973. There is an annual keyword index. It is also available online.

The Interdok Corporation, New York, publishes *Directory of published proceedings* (1964-); this appears monthly.

Vital statistics

A comprehensive guide to sources of medical statistical information in Britain has been published by Cowie (1986), and Hague (1986) has given some useful advice on handling statistical inquiries in a medical library. The chapter on 'Sources of vital statistics' in Welch and King (1985) provides an excellent account, and the Central Statistical Office publishes *Government statistics: a brief guide to sources*, annually, free of charge

World health statistics annual, Geneva, World Health Organization, 1952-
From 1939 to 1951 this appeared as Annual epidemiological and vital statistics. Contains life tables, changing mortality and morbidity rates, etc. for most countries of the world. In English and French.

Demographic yearbook. New York, 1948-
Prepared by the Statistical Office of the United Nations.

Contains statistics of population, nationality, mortality, marital state, divorce, and migration. In English and French. Supplemented by *Population and vital statistics report*.

Registrar General's statistical review of England and Wales 1837-1973, London, HMSO, 1838-1976.
Annual. The General Register Office also published *Weekly return of births and deaths, and infectious diseases and Quarterly return of births, deaths, and infectious diseases*. Similar statistics are provided by the Registrars General for Scotland and Northern Ireland. In 1970 the General Register Office and the Office of Social Surveys were merged to form the Office of Population Censuses and Surveys. The annual *Statistical review* was replaced in 1974 by the *OPCS reference series*, each series dealing with a particular aspect of vital statistics and supplemented by *OPCS Monitors*, designed to allow prompt publication of selected information (monthly, quarterly, or occasional). The *Quarterly return* was replaced by *Population trends* (quarterly) in 1974.

Selected list No. 56, London, HMSO.
Gives details of OPCS publications and is frequently revised. HMSO catalogues are now on BLAISE-LINE, the British Library's online system. It covers items listed since 1976 in daily, monthly and annual HMSO catalogues.

On the state of the public health, London, HMSO.
The annual report of the Chief Medical Officer of Health of the Department of Health and Social Security. Some statistics; particularly useful for topics of current interest.

Guide to official statistics, London, HMSO.
Compiled by the Central Statistical Office, this appears every two years. A guide to all official and some non-official statistics. Includes population, vital, and social statistics.

Annual abstract of statistics, London, HMSO.
Compiled by the Central Statistical Office. Covers summaries of UK statistics, usually over a ten-year span; includes population and vital statistics, mortality rates by age and cause, life tables, infectious disease notifications, etc.

Pharmaceutical literature

The *Guide to the literature of pharmacy and the pharmaceutical sciences* (Andrews, 1986) is an annotated bibliography of nearly 1,000 reference sources, standard texts, and periodicals. Extensive coverage of the literature on pharmacology and therapeutics is provided by Calam (1984). He discusses primary sources, abstracts and indexing services, reviews, monographs, pharmacopoeias, drug indexes, and legal requirements. Hands (1985) has given a full account of drug information services, including annotated lists of books and journals. A systematic account of the flow of pharmaceutical information has recently been published by Pickering (1990).

Following a recommendation of a working party set up by the (Royal) Pharmaceutical Society of Great Britain in 1974, drug information centres were established within each of the regional health authorities in the UK. National Poisons Centres had already been established; advice is available on a 24-hour basis from these centres in Belfast, Cardiff, Dublin, Edinburgh and London. An independent centre is based in Leeds.

British pharmacopoeia, 2 vols. London, Pharmaceutical Press, 1988.

The accepted legal standard in Britain and the Commonwealth countries for the drugs described in it. Publication is on the recommendation of the Medicines Commission. In due course the standards laid down in the *European pharmacopoeia* will become the accepted legal standards in Britain, replacing the corresponding standards in the *BP*.

Pharmaceutical codex, 11th edn., London, Pharmaceutical Press, 1979.

Formerly the *British pharmaceutical codex*, a supplement to the *BP*; now an encyclopaedia of information for all concerned with the preparation and use of drugs.

Martindale: Extra pharmacopoeia, 29th edn., London, Pharmaceutical Press, 1989.

Intended to provide information on the pharmaceutical and chemical properties, toxicity, contra-indications, actions and uses of all substances – official, unofficial, and proprietary. Contains over 6,000 monographs, and also abstracts

and references from recent literature. Includes a directory of manufacturers. Available online through DATA-STAR and DIALOG.
Martindale online: drug information thesaurus and user's guide (1984) contains the tailor-made thesaurus for the Martindale online databank.

European pharmacopoeia, Sainte-Ruffine, Maisonneuve.
Prepared under the auspices of the Council of Europe. The first edition in three volumes appeared in 1969-75. Publication of the second edition began in 1980, in loose-leaf form. Under the terms of a 1964 Convention it has been agreed that monographs published in the *BP* should become official in each member country from a specified date.

International pharmacopoeia. Pharmacopoeia internationalis, 3rd edn., Geneva, World Health Organization. Vol. 1: *General methods of analysis*, 1979; Vols. 2-3: *Quality specifications*, 1981-8.
Prepared by members of the WHO Expert Advisory Panel on the International Pharmacopoeia and Pharmaceutical Preparations, and other specialists. A collection of recommended methods and specifications not intended to have legal status as such in any country unless introduced for that purpose by appropriate legislation.

United States pharmacopoeia, Rockville, Md, US Pharmacopoeial Convention.
New edition every five years. Provides pharmacopoeial standards for drugs used in the USA.

British national formulary.
Published jointly by the British Medical Association and the Royal Pharmaceutical Society. Revised twice a year. A pocket-size guide to prescribing in hospital and general practice; the main guide to dispensing under the NHS. It includes an index of proprietary preparations and the non-proprietary equivalents.

Dental practitioners' formulary.
Similar to the *BNF*; deals with drugs used in dental surgery. For use under the NHS and published jointly by the BMA

and the RPS, in association with the British Dental Association.

British approved names 1986, London, Pharmaceutical Press.
Names devised or selected by the British Pharmacopoeia Commission. Gives pronunciation, systematic chemical definition and a general indication of action and use.

MIMS (Monthly index of medical specialities), London.
A monthly index of ethical proprietary preparations available for prescription in general practice in Britain. Entry is under proprietary name. Each issue supersedes its predecessor.

Association of the British Pharmaceutical Industry, *Data sheet compendium*, London, Datapharm Pubs. Ltd.
Annual. A compendium of data sheets submitted by British pharmaceutical houses. Gives information on presentation, uses, doses, contra-indications, etc. of pharmaceutical preparations.

Drug literature index, Amsterdam, Excerpta Medica.
Twice a month with annual cumulations. A published partial version of the computer tapes prepared for Excerpta Medica's DRUGDOC service. Indexes all articles containing a significant mention of drugs and related compounds. Includes generic names index, drug class index, trade names and author index.

Marler, E.E.J., *Pharmacological and chemical symbols*, 8th edn., Amsterdam, Excerpta Medica, 1985.
An alphabetical listing of non-proprietary names of drugs with a list of synonyms, chemical and alternative non-proprietary and proprietary names.

The Merck index. An encyclopedia of chemicals and drugs, 10th edn., Rahway, N.J., Merck, 1983.
A comprehensive index of information on the chemical and physical properties, doses and toxicities of about 10,000 compounds.

Meyler's Side effects of drugs, 11th edn., edited by M.N.G. Dukes. Amsterdam, Elsevier, 1988.
World-wide coverage of the literature on adverse drug

51

reactions. This work and *Side effects of drugs annual*, ed. M.N.G. Dukes are available online through the Excerpta Medica database SEDBASE.

Turner, P. and Vollans, G.N., *Drugs handbook*, 7th edn., London, Macmillan, 1987.
A guide to the uses, modes of action, and side effects of drugs.

7 Aids for writers and speakers

Results obtained in medical research are of little use unless they are made available in the form of publications or as papers read at meetings. The collection of references for the pursuit of a particular piece of research work or for a review of a particular subject is of little use to anyone except the person concerned unless destined for publication. References should be collected systematically, recorded properly, and verified before publication.

A bibliography is a comprehensive collection of references to the literature of the subject under consideration. Some writers use the term bibliography incorrectly to describe what is simply a collection of the references cited in a publication.

A bibliographical reference is a set of data describing a publication. It should be sufficiently detailed to permit identification without difficulty. A reference should not be included in a publication unless it is intended as confirmation of, or is relevant to, a statement by the writer of the publication, or unless it refers to further literature on the subject. 'Personal communications' and 'unpublished observations' should be mentioned in the text and not in the list of references.

When references are collected they are best recorded on separate slips or cards large enough to contain a few notes. In this form they can be filed systematically or arranged in the order required for publication. However, some people nowadays write straight on to a word processor (or at least file records on it). An excellent guide to the organization of personal files has been published by Roberts (1984).

Before preparing a paper for publication the writer should ascertain the requirements and style of the journal to which it is to be submitted. Most medical and scientific journals publish instructions to authors, either in each issue or occasionally (see Lane & Kammerer, below).

There are two principal methods of quoting references in the text of a paper. In January 1978 a group of editors from a number of major English-language biomedical journals met in Vancouver and drew up 'Uniform requirements for manuscripts submitted to biomedical journals', known as the Vancouver style. These were last revised in 1988 (International Committee, p.55). In the Vancouver style the references are numbered consecutively in the order in which they are first mentioned in the text and are listed in the same order at the end of the publication. Titles of journals given in references are abbreviated according to the style used in Index medicus. The Vancouver style also lays down requirements for the style of listing various other types of reference, for preparation of the manuscript, tables, illustrations, units of measurement, abbreviations, etc. This style is being used in an increasing number of journals.

The other common method of quoting references is by following the name of the author quoted with the date of publication, e.g. Smith (1988). The references are listed alphabetically by author at the end of the paper. This is the so-called Harvard method. Chernin (1988) has published a note on the history of this method of citation.

There are a number of publications offering advice on the preparation of papers for publication, on style in writing, speaking at meetings, etc. A selection of these is listed below. The reader is also referred to the list of basic reference works on pp. 40-52.

Baron, D.N. (ed.), *Units, symbols and abbreviations. A guide for biological and medical editors and authors,* 4th edn., London, Royal Society of Medicine, 1988.
    Originally based on recommendations of a working party set up at a conference of medical editors, London, 1968. Deals with metrication (SI units); principles for forming symbols and abbreviations: units, symbols, abbreviations; and conventions; layout of references.

Booth, V., *Writing a scientific paper*, 4th edn., London, Biochemical Society, 1977.

British Medical Journal, *How to do it*, 2nd edn., London, BMJ, 1985. *How to do it. 2*, London, BMJ, 1987.
 Eighty-four articles reprinted from the *British Medical Journal* covering a wide range of activities in which doctors might expect to engage in at some time in their career, such as giving a lecture, chairing a committee, keeping up with the literature, conducting an interview, writing a thesis, etc.

Calnan, J. & Barabas, A., *Writing medical papers*, London, Heinemann Medical, 1973.

Calnan, J. & Barabas, A., *Speaking at medical meetings*, 2nd edn., London, Heinemann Medical, 1981.

Ebel, H.F., Bleifert, C. & Russey, W.E., *The art of scientific writing: from student reports to professional publications in chemistry and related fields*, Weinheim, VCH Verlagsgesellschaft, 1987.

Fowler, H.W., *A dictionary of modern English usage*, 2nd edn., revised by Sir Ernest Gowers. Oxford, Clarendon Press, 1965.

Gowers, E., *The complete plain words*, London, HMSO, 1954.
 A reconstruction of two earlier works – *Plain words and ABC of plain words*, intended to improve style in English writing, particularly office documents.

Hawkins, C. & Sorgi, M. (eds.), *Research; how to plan, speak and write about it*, Berlin, Springer, 1985.
 A guide to planning research, searching the literature, preparing papers for publication, etc.

Huth, E.K., *How to write and publish papers*, Philadelphia, ISI Press, 1982.

International Committee of Medical Journal Editors, 'Uniform requirements for manuscripts submitted to biomedical journals'. Annals of Internal Medicine, 1988, **108**, 258-65; *British Medical Journal*, 1988, **296**, 401-5.

Lane, N.D. & Kammerer, K.L., *Writer's guide to medical periodicals*, Cambridge, Mass., Ballinger, 1975.

Provides detailed instructions on style requirements of over 300 general and research-orientated periodicals in the medical field; also includes information on the percentage of articles accepted by the various journals, and individual publishers' estimates of the time lag between manuscript submission and publication.

Lock, S., *Thorne's Better medical writing*, 2nd edn., London, Pitman, 1977.

O'Connor, M. & Woodford, F.P., *Writing scientific papers in English*, Amsterdam, Elsevier; London, Pitman, 1978.
Deals with all aspects of writing a paper, from planning to proof correcting.

Oxford dictionary for writers and editors, Compiled by the Oxford English Dictionary Department, Oxford, Clarendon Press, 1988.
The house style of the Oxford University Press. Gives guidance on the correct spelling and usage of everyday words and proper names, formation of plurals, abbreviations, etc.

Royal Society of London, *General notes on the preparation of scientific papers*, London, Royal Society, 1965.

Turabian, K.L., A manual for writers of research papers, theses and dissertations, London, Heinemann Medical, 1982.

8 Historical and biographical sources

Historical sources

There is an extensive literature on the history of medicine, both in books and periodicals, covering general medicine and its specialties. It is appropriate to mention a few sources and guides to the literature. A more detailed listing of historical and biographical material has been published by Freeman (1984).

A short history of medicine by Charles Singer and E.A. Underwood, 2nd edn., Oxford, Clarendon Press, 1962, is a very readable introduction to the subject. It includes a comprehensive list of references covering all branches of medicine.

One of the best single-volume publications, still regarded as the authoritative work in the English language, is F.H. Garrison's *Introduction to the history of medicine*, 4th edn., Philadelphia, Saunders, 1929, reprinted 1960. Garrison was a leading American authority on the history of medicine. The *Introduction* contains an extensive bibliography.

Sir William Osler's *Evolution of modern medicine*, New Haven, Yale University Press, 1921, is a good introduction to the subject.

Cecilia C. Mettler's *History of medicine, a correlative text*, Philadelphia, Blakiston, 1947, is arranged by broad subject sections. Each chapter includes a list of references for further reading. There are extensive name and subject indexes; the latter usefully includes dates of birth and death.

A history of medicine by Arturo Castiglioni was first published in Italian; it was translated and edited by E.B. Krumbhaar (2nd edn., New York, Aronson,1969). It is a good general survey arranged by periods and with useful bibliographies.

An excellent account of the subject from the seventeenth century onwards is provided by R.H. Shryock in his *Development of modern medicine* (Philadelphia, 1936, reprinted Madison, Univ. Wisconsin Press, 1979). More recently E. Ackerknecht has published *A short history of medicine*, Baltimore, Johns Hopkins Univ. Press, 1982. A.S. Lyons and R.J. Petrucelli's *Medicine, an illustrated history*, New York, Abrams, 1978, a folio-size volume, includes over 1,000 fine illustrations. The Encyclopedia of medical history, New York, McGraw Hill, 1985, was compiled by R.E. and M.P. McGrew.

Although space restricts the listing of foreign-language publications, mention must be made of the *Histoire générale de la médecine, de la pharmacie, de l'art dentaire et de l'art vétérinaire*, 3 vols., Paris, Michel, 1936-49. This magnificent work, beautifully illustrated, was written by experts in each branch of the subject under the general editorship of M.P.M. Laignel-Lavastine.

Henry Sigerist was a professional medical historian whose writings are always worth attention. His work, *The great doctors, a biographical history of medicine*, shows, through a series of biographies, the principal trends in the development of medicine. It was first published in German in 1932 and an English translation (London, Allen & Unwin, 1933) was reprinted in 1972.

Many anthologies are available, for example R.H. Major's *Classic descriptions of disease*, 3rd edn., Springfield, C.C. Thomas, 1945, and Logan Clendening's Source book of medical history, New York, Hoeber, 1942, reprinted (Dover), 1960. The latter contains extracts from the writings of 120 authors, translated where necessary, with historical and biographical notes. E.C. Kelly published five large volumes of *Medical classics*, Baltimore, 1936-41, Williams & Wilkins, which contain reprints of classical or historically important texts; English translations are added where necessary, and biographical notes and full bibliographies are provided.

Outstanding among the specialty anthologies is J.F. Fulton's *Selected readings in the history of physiology*. 2nd edn.,

Springfield, C.C. Thomas, 1966, with selections ranging from the works of Aristotle to those of twentieth-century writers.

Annotated lists of books and papers on medical history and biography, in both English and foreign languages, comprehensive and national, and covering periods and specialties, will be found in Blake and Roos (1967), see p. 40. An extensive list is provided in L.T. Morton's *A medical bibliography*, 4th edn., Aldershot, Gower, 1983. This is an annotated bibliography of 7800 items arranged under broad subject headings, recording the most important contributions to the development of medicine and related disciplines; it also includes a section on general histories of medicine, histories by period, locality and subject, and biographical sources. A useful adjunct to the second (1954) edition is Lee Ash's *Serial publications containing medical classics: an index of citations contained in Garrison-Morton*, 2nd edn., Bethany, Ct, Antiquarium, 1961. This is an alphabetic-chronological listing to the references to periodicals in the *Medical bibliography* – an invaluable aid to librarians building up collections of periodical papers of historical significance.

Books recording medical eponyms and eponymically-named syndromes are described on p. 42.

Joan S. Emmerson's *Translations of medical classics*, Newcastle upon Tyne, University Library Pub. No. 3, 1965, although not claiming to be comprehensive, lists a large number of English translations of classical texts published before 1900.

A mass of information on important contributions to medical knowledge is included in J.L. Thornton's *Medical books, libraries and collectors*, 3rd edn., edited by A. Besson, Aldershot, Gower, 1989.

The *Bibliography of the history of medicine* has been published by the National Library of Medicine since 1965. It is an annual, each fifth issue being a quinquennial cumulation. It is divided into three sections: biographies, a subject section arranged alphabetically under fairly general headings, and an author section.

Current work in the history of medicine (1954-) is published quarterly by the Wellcome Institute for the History of Medicine. It is a subject index to the literature and, besides articles from the perodical literature, it includes lists of new books. The Wellcome Institute's *Subject catalogue of the history of medicine and related sciences*, containing largely secondary literature, has been published in 18 volumes (three series – subject, topographical, and biographical) by Kraus International Publishers, Munich, 1980.

Biographical sources

Medical literature is well endowed with biographical material. Garrison (1928) described the available sources and outlined future prospects of medical biography. His essay lists general medical biographical collections and works that include biographical material as well as individual biographies. Payne (1970) has supplemented Garrison with a review of current medical biographical sources available, described some less well-known sources, and made suggestions for modern requirements.

The *Index-catalogue* (see p. 20) is a valuable source for references to biographical material, indexed under the names of biographees. The *Quarterly cumulative index medicus* (p. 23) indexes biographical articles from periodicals both under the names of individuals and under the headings BIOGRA-PHIES or OBITUARIES. The biographical section of the *Bibliography of the history of medicine* (see above) includes both medical and famous non-medical persons in its biographical section.

Isis cumulative bibliography, a bibliography of the history of science, formed from Isis Critical bibliographies, 1-100, 1913-71 includes (vol. 1-2, 1971, and vol. 1, 1981, London, Mansell) references to many medical men and women.

A bibliography of medical and biomedical biography, by L.T. Morton and R.J. Moore (Aldershot, Scolar, 1989) is based on J.L. Thornton's *Select bibliography of medical biography*, 2nd edn., London, Library Association, 1970, and although still restricted to works in English published after 1800, does include references to biochemists, geneticists, molecular biologists, and others who have made contributions of value to medicine. Appropriate entries from the *Biographical memoirs of fellows of the Royal Society* (p. 62), the *Biographical memoirs of the National Academy of Sciences*, Philadelphia, and the

Dictionary of scientific biography, are included, and archival collections are also noted in it.

The *Catalogue of biographies in the library of the New York Academy of Medicine*, Boston, Hall, 1960, contains 3450 entries referring mainly to separately-published biographies of physicians and scientists.

One of the best biographical works dealing with older material is August Hirsch's *Biographisches Lexikon der hervorragenden Ärzte aller Zeiten und Völker*, 6 vols., Vienna, Urban & Schwarzenberg, 1884-8. It includes biographical sketches of about 17,000 physicians and surgeons, listing principal publications and sources of additional information. A revised edition published in Berlin in 1929-35 incorporates the *Biographisches Lexikon hervorragender Ärzte des neunzehnten Jahrhunderts* by J. Pagel, 1901; this was reprinted in 1962 and again in 1988 (Basel, Karger). I. Fischer's *Biographisches Lexikon der hervorragenden Ärzte der letzten fünfzig Jahre*, 2 vols., Berlin, Urban & Schwarzenberg, 1932-3, also reprinted 1962, covers the period 1880-1930 and provides a supplement to Hirsch.

H.E. Sigerist's *Great doctors*, London, Allen & Unwin, 1933 (reprinted 1972) contains about 50 short biographies ranging from the period of Ancient Egyptian medicine to modern times.

William Macmichael's *The gold-headed cane* was first published anonymously in 1827. It has been reprinted several times, most recently in 1968 (Royal College of Physicians). Autobiographical in form, it recounts the adventures of a gold-headed cane that came, in turn, into the possession of some seventeenth- and eighteenth-century British physicians (Radcliffe, Mead, Askew, William and David Pitcairn, and Baillie) and was then retired to a glass case in the library of the Royal College of Physicians of London, where it remains today. Besides providing good biographies of the various owners of the cane, the book gives interesting information on the condition of medicine in England at that time.

William Munk's *Roll of the Royal College of Physicians of London*, 2nd edn., 3 vols., London, The College, 1878, contains short biographical sketches of 1,723 fellows and licentiates of the College from its foundation in 1518 up to

1825. Several supplements bring the Roll to 1988. It is a good starting point for biographical information on British physicians, eminent or otherwise.

A similar service to British surgeons was performed by V.G. Plarr. *Plarr's Lives of the fellows of the Royal College of Surgeons of England*, Bristol, for The College, 1930, was published in two volumes and includes references to publications, portraits and sources of additional information. Several supplements have since been published, the most recent being in 1988, bringing the record up to the year 1982.

The Royal College of Obstetricians and Gynaecologists is a comparatively recent foundation (1929) but it already has a biographical record in Sir John Peel's *Lives of the fellows of the Royal College of Obstetricians and Gynaecologists 1929-1969*, London, Heinemann Medical, 1970.

The Royal Society of London publishes an annual volume of *Biographical memoirs of fellows of the Royal Society*. This was begun in 1955 as a continuation of *Obituary notices of fellows of the Royal Society*, vols. 1-9, 1932-54. The *Biographical memoirs* are lengthy, authoritative articles usually written from personal knowledge of the biographee, with a bibliography of his writings and a portrait.

Notable names in medicine and surgery, by Hamilton Bailey and W.J. Bishop, 4th edn., ed. Harold Ellis, London, H.K. Lewis, 1983, contains short biographical notes on about 80 physicians and surgeons whose names are perpetuated in medical terminology (e.g. 'Erb's palsy', 'Unna's paste', 'Heberden's nodes', etc.)

Brief biographical details of contemporary medical men may be found in *Who's who* and the *Medical directory* and their foreign equivalents. The British *Medical directory* has appeared annually since 1845. It gives the name, address, qualifications, past and present appointments and up to three publications of each entrant. It also has information on hospitals, medical schools and postgraduate institutions, medical societies, etc. in Britain.

The *Medical register*, issued annually since 1859 under the authority of the General Medical Council, publishes the name, address and medical qualifications of every person fully or provisionally registered to practise in Great Britain, including practitioners eligible by virtue of recognized qualifications obtained abroad.

Dentists in Britain are recorded in the annual *Dentists register*, an alphabetical listing with sections for the Commonwealth and for those holding foreign diplomas. Its maintenance is the responsibility of the General Dental Council.

One of the best sources for American medical biography is the *Dictionary of American medical biography*, by H.A. Kelly and W.L. Burrage, New York, Appleton, 1928, which is really the third edition of Kelly's *Cyclopedia of American medical biography*, Philadelphia, 1912. A more up-to-date source is the *Dictionary of American medical biography*, ed. by M. Kaufman et al., 2 vols., Westport, Conn., Greenwood Press, 1984.

The 16-volume *Dictionary of scientific biography*, ed. by C.C. Gillispie, New York, Charles Scribner's Sons, 1970-80, consists of over 5,000 lengthy biographies contributed by professional historians of science and medicine. The *World who's who in science*, first published in 1968; is a biographical dictionary containing some 30,000 short sketches of scientists from antiquity to the present.

The cumulated subject indexes of *Chemical abstracts* and *Biological abstracts* are worth consulting for references to biographies and obituaries of chemists, biologists, physiologists and biochemists.

9 Audio-visual aids

Audio-visual aids (non-book materials) are an important supplement to books and lectures in medical education. They include films, film-strip, slides, audio-tapes, videos and video-disks, models, etc. One advantage that audio-visual aids have over lectures is that the user can re-run a tape or slide sequence to repeat something missed or incompletely understood. Here the subject can only be dealt with briefly; for up-to-date information the reader is referred to the Audio-visual column regularly contributed to Health libraries review by Margaret C. Stewart (formerly Jones). See also Jones (1984, 1986) and Birnhack (1988)

Sources

The Graves Medical Audiovisual Library was established in 1957 with the object of helping general practitioners to keep up to date. At first it had the backing of the Royal College of General Practitioners; now it is an independent charity. Material is loaned on a subscription basis. A new complete catalogue of the tape-slides, videos and other material available in the library is published every two years, with updating lists distributed every six months. A National Medical Slide Bank was established at the Graves Library a few years ago and now numbers over 10,000 slides. A catalogue of this slide bank is also available. The address of the Graves Medical Audiovisual Library is Holly House, 220 New London Road, Chelmsford, Essex CM2 9BJ.

The National Audio Visual Aids Library, The George Building, Normal College, Holyhead Road, Bangor, Gwynedd LL57 2PZ was established by the Educational Foundation for Visual Aids in 1949. It is probably the largest educational film library in the UK. Its catalogue, *Audiovisual aids, Part 6 (ii), Human biology, hygiene and health teacher education*, published in 1973, with supplements to 1979, aims to provide one combined list of audio-visual material for use in schools, colleges and training centres.

The University of London Audio-Visual Centre was established in 1968 to further the co-ordinated use of audio-visual materials and methods by advice and help, to produce television recordings, films and other audio-visual aids to teaching and learning, and to establish a library of such material. Its catalogue, which includes medical material, is regularly updated. The Centre is at North Wing Studios, Senate House, Malet Street, London WC1E 7JZ.

Health education index is published every two to three years by Edsall Publishing Group, Home and Law Publishing Ltd, Greater London House, Hampstead Road, London NW1 3YP. It lists a wide variety of types of programmes for health education, arranged by subject and subdivided by format. The ninth edition covers 1987-8.

A Video Library of Surgery and Medicine is being assembled by the Royal Society of Medicine in association with the Royal College of Surgeons of England. The first six videos were published in 1984 and many others have appeared since. They may be hired or bought from Macmillan Medical Video Publications, Brunel Road, Houndsmill, Basingstoke RG2 2BR.

Although the United Kingdom has an inter-library lending system of outstanding efficiency for printed material, the same cannot be said of non-print media. Measures being taken towards its improvement are described by Cornish (1987), who discusses the paucity of bibliographic sources for audio-visual materials and the problems still outstanding.

Information

The British Universities Film and Video Council, 55 Greek Street, London W1V 5LR runs an information service. Its *British Universities Film and Video Council catalogue*, published every two years, is probably the largest catalogue of audio-visual material now in existence, with over 5,500 entries (*Health libraries review*, 1986, **3** 186) several hundred of which are relevant to the medical field. Its 1989 catalogue is available on microfiche. It also publishes *Distributors' index* which lists the catalogues of individual distributors, including many on medical topics. The Council's *Viewfinder* (previously *BUFC Newsletter*), appears three times a year and, besides reporting the work of the Council, deals with audio-visual material on higher education in general. In collaboration with the University of London Audio-Visual Centre (see above) the BUFVC also publishes *Videodisc newsletter* three times a year.

An international guide to locating audio-visual information has been published by Jones (1986).

Among the services offered by the Educational Foundation for Visual Aids are the maintenance and repair of almost any equipment from video systems and computers to slide projectors, hire of audio-visual and video presentation systems, sales of audio-visual equipment and hire and sales of educational films and videos. Jones (1987) gives a list of the Educational Foundation's offices from which information may be obtained regarding its products and repair services.

An excellent series of user specifications for equipment (USPECs) is published by the Council for Educational Technology, 3 Devonshire Street, London W1.

Catalogues

Besides the catalogues produced by bodies mentioned above, some other sources should be mentioned.

The *Educational film video locator of the consortium of university film centers and R.R. Bowker*, 3rd edn., New York, Bowker, 1986, lists 48,000 selected film and video titles. Entries are annotated and arranged alphabetically by title and subject. It is updated every three years.

British medicine (monthly) includes a classified list of non-book material.

Concord Video and Film Council, 201 Felixstowe Road, Ipswich IP3 9BJ deals with documentation, animated films, and feature-length productions concerned with contemporary issues, both at home and abroad. Films are selected primarily to promote discussion for instruction and training in schools and colleges and in the health service and other social services. Its latest catalogue is for 1989-91; supplements are published as required and are free to subscribers. The catalogue is arranged in alphabetical order, with subject index. All its programmes are available for hire and many for sale.

The Royal Society of Medicine Film and Television Unit has a catalogue of available video titles. It is obtainable from the Unit at Box 882, Worcester WR6 6YH.

Oxford Educational Resources Ltd, 197 Botley Road, Oxford OX2 OHE distributes a great deal of material originating from universities and teaching hospitals in Britain and the USA as well as the programmes formerly available from Camera Talks Ltd.

Health sciences audiovisuals is a quarterly catalogue published by the National Library of Medicine in microfiche.

Online sources

HELPIS (Higher Education Learning Programmes Information Service) is the British Universities Film and Video Council's database available through BLAISE. It includes the contents of the current *BUFVC catalogue* plus new material accumulating for the next edition. Search may be made by subject, title, format, language, country of origin, producer, or year of publication.

AVMARC (AudioVisual MAchine Readable Catalogue) is the British Library's online search service for audio-visual materials. It aims to include as much as possible of such material available within the UK. Search may be made via BLAISE by subject, title, or format, by users with their own terminals, or by post from the British Library.

AVLINE (Audiovisual Online), produced by the National Library of Medicine, Bethesda, Md, USA, has bibliographical records of all types of medical and dental audio-visual material from 1976 to date. Access is through BLAISE-LINK and MEDLARS. *Health sciences audiovisuals* is a quarterly printout of everything on AVLINE; it is published by the NLM in microfiche.

AV-ONLINE is the world's largest database of instructive material, including films, film-strips, video-strips, video-cassettes, slide sets, overhead transparencies, records, etc. on all subjects. It is run by the National Information Center for Educational Media, Access Innovations Inc., P.O. Box 40130,

Albuquerque, New Mexico 87196, USA. Access is through DIALOG.

Periodical publications

British medicine, Viewfinder and *Videodisc newsletter* have already been mentioned. The *Journal of audiovisual media in medicine*, London (quarterly) publishes original articles, book reviews, notes on new equipment and methods and journal abstracts dealing with the application and use of audio-visual techniques. In the United States, the quarterly *Journal of biocommunication* San Francisco, performs a similar service.

Audiovisual librarian is a quarterly publication by the Audio-visual Groups of Aslib and the Library Association. Although the emphasis of *AV user* (Maclaren, 1988-) is very much on technical matters, it does include a monthly listing of new catalogues, both for equipment and audio-visual programmes. It is also a response magazine, i.e. it is sent only to those who indicate an active interest in audio-visuals by seeking further information on published items.

The National Interactive Video Centre, 24-32 Stephenson Way, London NW1 2HD has published the quarterly *Interactive* since 1986.

10 Biomedical library facilities in Britain

Information about over 600 medical libraries in Britain is contained in the *Directory of medical and health care libraries in the United Kingdom and Republic of Ireland* (Linton, 1986). A useful *Guide to government departments and other libraries and information bureaux* is published by the Science Reference Library and revised about once a year.

Although the use of the libraries mentioned below is sometimes restricted to their members, reference facilities are usually granted to other *bona fide* users on application to the librarian.

Collections of medical books have existed in Britain since the early Middle Ages. Since that time the medical corporations and societies, the universities, the medical schools and research institutions have all contributed to the development of medical libraries, and Britain today is a rich storehouse of medical literature. Its greatest concentration is in London where several royal colleges, the Royal Society of Medicine, the Wellcome Institute for the History of Medicine, the British Medical Association, the postgraduate medical institutes and the medical schools provide a collection of medical literature probably unsurpassed anywhere else in the country.

The medical corporations

The medical corporations were established for the purpose of raising the standard of their profession and increasing their knowledge of it. They are empowered to grant recognized diplomas to suitably qualified persons. They comprise the royal colleges of physicians and surgeons of London, Edinburgh, Glasgow and Dublin, several other recently-established specialist royal colleges, and the Society of Apothecaries.

The Royal College of Physicians of London was founded in 1518 through the efforts of Thomas Linacre, whose books formed the nucleus of its library. Unfortunately the College building was destroyed in the Great Fire of London and all but 140 of the books perished. Bequests from fellows of the College provided an important source of additions to the library for many years but it was not until the nineteenth century that serious attention was given to its development. Today it contains about 50,000 volumes, including some incunabula, and a magnificent collection of 10,000 engraved portraits and photographs. It is available for reference to fellows and all *bona fide* research workers.

The Royal College of Physicians of Edinburgh was founded in 1681 and immediately began to build up a library. Today it contains over 72,000 volumes, including 880 sets of current periodicals. It is available to members of the College and others.

Although the Royal College (formerly Faculty) of Physicians and Surgeons of Glasgow was founded in 1599, it was not until a hundred years later that it began the formation of a library. It now has a good modern library supported by a rich historical collection, together totalling about 200,000 volumes and 360 sets of current journals. It is available to staff and other readers.

The Royal College of Surgeons of Edinburgh received its present title in 1778, although its history goes back to 1505. Its library was started around 1696 but in 1763 the Surgeons found themselves in financial difficulties and were obliged to rent their premises to others. They were hard pressed to find space for the library, which eventually passed into the possession of the University of Edinburgh. However, in 1845 the fortunes of the College had sufficiently improved for it to begin to form its present library. Today it possesses about 32,000 volumes. It is open only to fellows of the College and other bona fide researchers

The Royal College of Surgeons of England traces its origin to the formation of the Company of Barber Surgeons in 1540. The barbers parted company with the surgeons in 1745 and disposed of the library six years later. The College was re-formed under its present title in 1800 and the systematic collection of books began in the new College in 1807. At the present time it contains about 160,000 volumes and takes 600 current journals. It possesses an extensive collection of engraved portraits. It is available to fellows and diplomates of the College and to other *bona fide* users on application to the librarian.

The Royal College of Surgeons in Ireland, Dublin, began to form a library as soon as it was founded in 1784. The library is rich in historical and archival material in addition to its modern collection of textbooks and journals. Its stock is about 53,000 volumes and it takes 400 current journals. A new building for the library is under construction; this will also accommodate the library of the Royal College of Physicians of Ireland (1654).

The Royal College of Obstetricians and Gynaecologists has been in existence since 1929. It is developing a specialist library of both historical and current works. It is available to members of the College and to suitably qualified persons for reference.

The Royal College of General Practitioners was established in 1952. Its medical recording service, now the Graves Medical Audiovisual Library, was inaugurated in 1957 (p. 64). It maintains a good library and offers a bibliographical service on general practice publications (p. 27).

The medical societies

Unlike the medical corporations, medical societies in Britain do not have the power to grant qualifications. Their members meet to share common interests and to exchange experiences. Some of the societies maintain fine libraries for the use of their members.

The Medical Society of London was established in 1773. In 1800 it purchased the valuable private library of its president, James Sims, amounting to some 6,000 volumes. Sims was first elected president in 1786 and his constant re-election to that office year after year eventually led, in 1805, to the secession of a number of discontented members. They formed a new society, the (Royal) Medical and Chirurgical Society of London, now the Royal Society of Medicine. The Medical Society of London disposed of its library a few years ago, much of its contents passing to the Wellcome Institute for the History of Medicine.

Prominent among the aims of the Medical and Chirurgical Society was the development of an extensive professional library, an objective vigorously pursued for the next hundred years. By 1907 it had a splendid library, and in that year it was amalgamated with 14 other societies concerned mainly with medical specialties and was renamed the Royal Society of Medicine. These other societies added their own specialist collections to the library, which today contains some 600,000 volumes and 2,000 sets of current periodicals. Both with regard to stock and to the services it offers its members, the Royal Society of Medicine has the best medical library in Britain. Membership is not restricted to those holding medical qualifications; in 1956 the Society formed a Library (Scientific Research) Section to make the library and other services available to industrial organizations, government departments, publishers and private bodies associated with medical problems. Non-members may use it on the introduction of a fellow.

Medical societies have been active in the provinces, notably in Liverpool and Manchester. The Liverpool Medical Institution was founded about 1773 by local medical practitioners as a reading club. It is now the centre of medical life in Liverpool and maintains a good library. The Manchester Medical Library dates from 1834 and in 1931 became an integral part of the medical library of Manchester University.

The British Medical Association was founded in 1832 as the Provincial Medical and Surgical Association, for the purpose of collecting useful knowledge and publishing transactions. In its early years it was preoccupied with medico-political matters and did not begin the formation of a library for its members until 1887. A few years ago much of its older stock was transferred to the library of the Wellcome Institute for the History of Medicine and it now concentrates on modern literature and special services to its members. Its present stock is about 30,000 volumes and 1000 sets of current periodicals. Most medical practitioners in Britain belong to the BMA. Its library is open to members and to others at the discretion of the librarian.

The British Dental Association Library was founded in 1920. Its stock includes 20,000 volumes and 200 sets of current journals, and it has a collection of early dental literature. It is open to members; others may use it for reference.

The Royal Pharmaceutical Society of Great Britain possesses an outstanding collection on the subject. The Society was founded in 1842 and now has about 65,000 volumes and takes 500 current journals. Its historical collection includes many herbals and London, Edinburgh and Dublin pharmacopoeias.

The teaching institutions

The first chair of medicine in Britain was established at Aberdeen University in 1495. At present 19 British universities offer medical teaching and maintain medical libraries.

The two oldest hospitals in London, St Bartholomew's and St Thomas', had libraries as early as 1667, although these were not confined to medical books. In London and other large cities and towns numerous general hospitals were established by local philanthropy during the eighteenth century, to be followed by special hospitals in the nineteenth. These two centuries were marked by an important development in medical education – the foundation of medical schools attached to teaching hospitals. Some of these schools absorbed, or were developed from, private schools. They formed libraries that are today the backbone of undergraduate medical teaching. In London there are ten medical schools, all attached to large general hospitals and forming part of the University of London.

In order to improve postgraduate teaching facilities in London the (Royal) Postgraduate Medical School was established in 1935 and was attached to Hammersmith Hospital, a large general hospital. Further improvement and a measure of co-ordination followed the formation of the British Postgraduate Medical Federation by the University of London in 1945. The Federation established specialist medical institutes for teaching and research, with good specialized libraries run by experienced librarians. Although they are rather young libraries they already play an important part in medical education and research. An outstanding postgraduate institution is the London School of Hygiene and Tropical Medicine, originating in 1899 as the London School of Tropical Medicine. Its library has 86,000 volumes and owns special collections associated with Manson and Ross. It receives about 1,000 periodicals currently, some of them via the Bureau of Hygiene and Tropical Diseases, which is housed in the School and is responsible for producing *Abstracts on hygiene* and the *Tropical diseases bulletin.*

Outside of London, Aberdeen, Edinburgh (which has a modern central medical library with 72,000 volumes), Manchester, Birmingham, Bristol, Glasgow, Cardiff and other cities have notable medical collections within their universities.

In the early part of the twentieth century the provision of library facilities for nurses was retarded by the paucity of literature on the subject. The first professional library for nurses was opened in Edinburgh by the Royal College of Nursing in 1916. In 1921 the College established its London library, the most important nursing collection in the country which now contains some 45,000 volumes and 220 sets of current periodicals.

The research institutions

Government-sponsored medical research in Britain followed the establishment of the Medical Research Council in 1913. The formation of its principal library at the National Institute for Medical Research was delayed until 1919 owing to the First World War. Today this library is the leading medical research library in the country, with a stock of 75,000 volumes, 500 current journals, and a considerable reprint collection. It serves the scientific staff of the Council working at the Institute and in other Council establishments throughout the country.

An important recent (1970) addition to the Council's research institutes is the Clinical Research Centre at Northwick Park Hospital, Harrow, which, as its name suggests, is particularly well stocked with material on clinical medicine. It has about 45,000 volumes and takes 650 current journals. Its librarian has published a detailed account of the publications of the Medical Research Council (Wade, 1989).

Other research institutes, such as the Central Public Health Laboratory, the National Institute for Biological Standards and Control, and the Imperial Cancer Research Fund, have valuable specialized collections. Much research is carried out in the postgraduate institutes, to which reference has already been made, and of course in the universities.

Industrial pharmaceutical libraries are comparatively recent. The pharmaceutical houses, however, have financial resources that permit the development of good libraries, and the drive and pressure behind their research demand first-class, efficient and resourceful library staff. These libraries serve the interests not only of research but also of the medical information and advisory services, manufacturing, and industrial health and welfare.

Other libraries

One of the best collections of medico-historical material owes its formation to the generosity of Sir Henry Wellcome (1853-1936), the pharmaceutical chemist. It was begun by Wellcome in 1895 as a private collection and was opened to the public in 1949. The library of the Wellcome Institute for the History of Medicine contains over 400,000 volumes, 10,000 manuscripts, more than 600 incunabula, 75,000 autograph letters, 60,000 pamphlets, and about 400 sets of current periodicals. It produces the quarterly *Current work in the history of medicine*, which lists all important books and articles. Several printed catalogues of the contents of the library have been published.

The principal government library concerned with medicine is that of the Department of Health and Social Security, founded in 1834. It is concerned with all aspects of state medicine and public health and welfare. It takes about 2,000 current periodicals and possesses 210,000 volumes. It has an extensive collection of annual reports of local authority medical officers. It maintains DHSS-data, a computerized database by means of which it produces several journals (see p. 31). It is available to staff and to others by appointment. For an account of the publications of the DHSS, see Shrigley (1989).

The Office of Population Censuses and Surveys was established in 1970 by the merger of the General Register Office and the Government Social Survey Department. Its library has a comprehensive range of British and foreign publications

75

concerned with population and medical statistics, censuses, social surveys, etc. It takes 350 current periodicals covering its fields of interest (see p. 48).

Since the early 1960s several hundred postgraduate centres have been established in Britain, mainly in non-teaching hospitals, to provide suitable facilities for postgraduate teaching of hospital staff and general medical and dental practitioners, and to cater for consultants, junior hospital staff and general practitioners who wish to meet and discuss problems of common interest. Standards of library provision in these centres vary considerably; most have only small libraries. In some cases a regional organization has been or is being developed covering all libraries within the area administered by the Regional Health Authority and backed by the resources of the associated university medical school.

The metropolitan libraries of London, by agreement, collect between them all books published in Britain and those foreign publications that are within their means. Under this scheme Westminster City Libraries maintain a medical collection at the Public Library, Marylebone Road, London NW1, and other libraries may take advantage of this collection through their inter-library loan facilities.

The British Library

The British Library was established in 1973 by the amalgamation of the library departments of the British Museum, National Central Library, National Lending Library for Science and Technology, and other organizations. It now contains over 16,000,000 volumes (books, periodicals, maps, manuscripts, etc.) and 1,000,000 disks.

The British Library Document Supply Centre at Boston Spa, Wetherby, West Yorkshire, has 380 miles of shelving and is the largest library in the world devoted to the supply of documents. It is the national centre for library inter-lending in the UK and between the UK and overseas countries. It supplies material only to other libraries, not direct to individuals. Applications for loans and photocopies are made through libraries registered as borrowers. Loan request forms are sold in books of 50, the cost of which covers postage on loans to borrowers.

The British Library's Science Reference and Information Service has two reading rooms in London; the Reading Room in Kean Street, Aldwych, houses literature on the life and earth sciences, while the Reading Room in Chancery Lane contains literature on physical sciences, engineering and patents. Both are open to the public.

The British Library receives several thousand medical titles out of a total of about 72,000 current serials taken. The *Current list of serials* published by the Document Supply Centre records titles but not holdings, and it is frequently updated. *Serials in the British Library*, a quarterly listing with annual cumulations, gives title, place of publication, date of commencement, and frequency; it is published by the British National Bibliographic Service of the British Library, London.

References

Andrews, T., *Guide to the literature of pharmacy and the pharmaceutical sciences*, Littleton, Col., Libraries Unlimited, 1986.

Birnhack, J., *Audiovisual resources in a hospital medical library: their organization and management*, London, Mansell, 1988.

Blake, J.B. & Roos, C., *Medical reference works 1679-1966*, Chicago, Medical Library Association, 1967.

Brandon, A.N. & Hill, D.R., 'Selected list of books and journals for the small medical library', *Bulletin of the Medical Library Association*, **77**, 1989, 139-69.

Calam, D.H., 'Pharmacology and therapeutics', in Morton, L.T. & Godbolt, S. (eds.), *Information sources in the medical sciences*, 3rd edn., London, Butterworths, pp. 188-207, 1984.

Carmel, M. (ed.), *Medical librarianship*, London, Library Association, 1981

Chernin, E., 'The "Harvard system": a mystery dispelled', *British medical journal*, **297**, 1988, 1062-3.

Clark, M.V., *Medical reference works 1679-1966. Supplement I, 1967-68*, Chicago, Medical Library Association, 1970.

Cooke, R., Gillespie, I. & Hartley, B., 'Training for Library Association chartering in health-care libraries. III', *Health libraries review*, **6**, 1989, 25-8.

Cornish, G.P. 'Interlending of audio-visual materials: a neglected national resource for medical and health libraries', *Health libraries review*, **4**, 1987, 164-71.

Cowie, A., 'Medical statistical information: a guide to sources', *Health libraries review*, **3**, 1986, 203-21.

Dalby, A.K., *Medical abstracts and indexes 1975*, Cambridge University Library, 1975.

Dannatt, R., 'Primary sources of information', in Morton, L.T. & Godbolt, S., (eds.), *Information sources in the medical sciences*, 3rd edn., London, Butterworths, pp. 17-43, 1984.

Dannatt, R. & Liepa, D., 'Serials', in Carmel, M., *Medical librarianship*, London, Library Association, pp. 82-99, 1981.

Darling, L. (ed.), *Handbook of medical library practice*, 4th edn., 3 vols., Chicago, Medical Library Association, 1982-8.

Fox, T., *Crisis in communication: the functions and future of medical journals*, London, Athlone Press, 1965.

Freeman, E.J., 'Historical, biographical and bibliographical sources', in Morton, L.T. & Godbolt, S., *Information sources in the medical sciences*, 3rd edn., London, Butterworths, pp. 463-90, 1984.

Garfield, E., 'Science Citation Index – a new dimension in indexing', *Science*, **144**, 1964, 649-54.

Garfield, E., 'Citation indexing for studying science', *Nature*, **227**, 1970, 669-71.

Garrison, F.H., 'Available sources and future prospects of medical biography', *Bulletin of the New York Academy of Medicine*, **4**, 1928, 586-607.

Garrison, F.H., 'The medical and scientific periodicals of the 17th and 18th centuries', *Bulletin of the Institute of the History of Medicine*, **2**, 1934, 285-343.

Godbolt, S., 'At the end of all our work is a patient', *Library Association record*, **79**, 1977, 86-9.

Hague, H., 'Standard reference sources', in Morton, L.T. & Godbolt, S., *Information sources in the medical sciences*, 3rd edn., London, Butterworths, pp. 70-89, 1984.

Hague, H., 'Handling statistical enquiries in the medical library – some practical examples', *Aslib proceedings*, **38**, 1986, 168-75.

Hands, D.E., 'Drug information services', in Welch, J. & King, T.A. *Searching the medical literature*, London, Chapman & Hall, pp. 73-103, 1985.

Hewlett, J., 'Training for Library Association chartering in health-care libraries', *Health libraries review*, **5**, 1988a, 181-8.

Hewlett, J., 'Pre-registration training in health-care libraries. II. Progress assessment check-list', *Health libraries review*, **5**, 1988b, 237-45.

Howard-Jones, N., 'Our medical literature – then and now', *British journal of medical education*, **7**, 1973, 70-85.

Jenkins, S., *Medical libraries: a user guide*, London, British Medical Association, 1987.

Jones, M.C., 'Audio-visual materials', in Morton, L.T. & Godbolt, S., (eds.), *Information sources in the medical sciences*, 3rd edn., London, Butterworths, pp. 491-511, 1984.

Jones, M.C., *International guide to locating audio-visual information in the health sciences*, Aldershot, Gower, 1986.

Jones, M.C., 'The Educational Foundation for Visual Aids', *Health libraries review*, **4**, 1987, 260.

Karel, L., 'Selection of journals for *Index Medicus*: a historical review', *Bulletin of the Medical Library Association*, **55**, 1967, 259-78.

Kronick, D.A., 'The Fielding H. Garrison list of medical and scientific periodicals of the 17th and 18th centuries: addenda and corrigenda', *Bulletin of the history of medicine*, **32**, 1958, 456-74.

Kronick, D.A., *A history of scientific and technical periodicals*, 2nd ed., Metuchen, Scarecrow Press, 1976.

LeFanu, W.R., *British periodicals of medicine: a chronological list*, Baltimore, Johns Hopkins Press, 1938. Reprinted from *Bulletin of the Institute of the History of Medicine*, **5**, 1937, 735-61, 827-55; **6**, 1938, 614-48. Revised edition, 1640-1899, Oxford, Wellcome Unit of the History of Medicine, 1984.

Linton, W.D. (comp.), *Directory of medical and health care libraries in the United Kingdom and the Republic of Ireland*, 6th edn., London, Library Association, 1986. [7th edn., comp. Wright, D.J., 1990, in press.]

Lyon, E. *Online medical databases 1989*, London, Aslib, 1988.

Martindale, *Martindale online: drug information thesaurus and user's guide*, London, Pharmaceutical Press, 1984.

Mills, J., *A modern outline of library classification*, London, Chapman & Hall, 1960.

Morton, L.T., *A medical bibliography (Garrison and Morton): an annotated check-list of texts illustrating the history of medicine*, 4th edn., Aldershot, Gower, 1983.

Morton, L.T., 'The growth of medical periodical literature', in Thornton, J.L., *Medical books, libraries and collectors*. 3rd edn., ed, A. Besson. Aldershot, Gower, 1990, pp. 221-38.

Morton, L.T. & Godbolt, S. (eds.), *Information sources in the medical sciences*, 3rd edn., London, Butterworths, 1984.

Orr, R.H. & Leeds, A.A., 'Biomedical literature: volume, growth and other characteristics', *Federation proceedings*, **23**, 1964, 1310-31.

Payne, L.M., 'Materials for medical biography', *Proceedings of Third International Congress of Medical Librarianship, Amsterdam, 5-9 May 1969*. Amsterdam, Excerpta Medica, 1970, 251-7.

Pickering, W.R. (ed.), *Information sources in pharmaceuticals*, London, Butterworths, 1989.

Porter, J.R., 'The scientific journal – 300th anniversary', *Bacteriological reviews*, **28**, 1964, 211-30.

Richmond, J.S., *Medical reference works 1679-1966. Supplement II, 1969-72; Supplement III, 1973-74*, Chicago, Medical Library Association, 1973-5.

Roberts, D.C., 'The organization of personal index files', in Morton, L.T. & Godbolt, S. (eds.) *Information sources in the medical sciences*, 3rd edn., London, Butterworths, pp. 512-22, 1984. Rogers, F.B. & Adams, S., 'The Army Medical Library's publication program', *Texas reports on biology and medicine*, **8**, 1950, 271-300.

Roper, F.W. & Boorkman, J., *Introduction to reference sources in the health sciences*, Chicago, Medical Library Association, 1980.

Shadrake, A.M. 'British medical periodicals, 1938-61', *Bulletin of the Medical Library Association*, **51**, 1963, 181-96.

Shrigley, S.M., 'Extending access to DHSS publications', *Health libraries review*, **6**, 1989, 124-7.

Spanier, L.M., *Biomedical serials 1950-1960*, Washington, D.C., U.S. Dept. of Health, Education, and Welfare, 1962.

Sutherland, F.M. 'Indexes, abstracts, bibliographies and reviews', in Morton. L.T. & Godbolt, S. (eds.), *Information sources in the medical sciences,* 3rd edn., London, Butterworths, 1984, pp. 44-69.

Wade, J., 'Publications of the Medical Research Council', *Health libraries review,* 6, 1989, 76-82.

Welch, J. & King, T.A., *Searching the medical literature. A guide to printed and online sources,* London, Chapman & Hall, 1985.

Index

84

85

87